CODEINE DIARY

CODEINE DIARY

A MEMOIR

TOM ANDREWS

LITTLE, BROWN AND COMPANY
BOSTON ■ NEW YORK ■ TORONTO ■ LONDON

First Edition

The author is grateful for permission to include the following previously copyrighted material:

Excerpt from "Litany" from *As We Know,* by John Ashbery. Copyright © 1979 by John Ashbery. Reprinted by permission of Viking Penguin, a division of Penguin Books USA, Inc.

Article from *Charleston Daily Mail* reprinted by permission of *Charleston Daily Mail.*

Excerpt from *The Letters of Emily Dickinson,* edited by Thomas H. Johnson, Cambridge, Mass.: The Belknap Press of Harvard University Press. Copyright © 1958, 1986 by the President and Fellows of Harvard College. Reprinted by permission of the publishers.

Letters by Norris McWhirter reprinted by permission of Guinness Publishing.

Letter by William Stafford reprinted by permission of Kim Stafford, the Estate of William Stafford.

Excerpt from "Vacancy in the Park" from *Collected Poems,* by Wallace Stevens. Copyright 1954 by Wallace Stevens. Reprinted by permission of Alfred A. Knopf, Inc.

Portions of this book appeared earlier in *Field, Harper's,* and *The Hemophiliac's Motorcycle,* by Tom Andrews, reprinted by permission of the University of Iowa Press.

LIBRARY OF CONGRESS CATALOGING-IN-PUBLICATION DATA

Andrews, Tom.
    Codeine diary : a memoir / by Tom Andrews. — 1st ed.
        p.   cm.
    ISBN 0-316-04244-7
    1. Andrews, Tom — Health.   2. Hemophiliacs — United States —
Biography.   3. Poets, American — Biography.   I. Title.
RC642.A54   1998
362.1′961572′0092 — dc21
[B]   97-17248

COVER DESIGN JEANNE ABBOUD

MV-NY

10 9 8 7 6 5   4 3 2 1

*Published simultaneously in Canada by Little, Brown &
Company (Canada) Limited*

PRINTED IN THE UNITED STATES OF AMERICA

To the memory of my brother
JOHN HOWARD ANDREWS
1956 – 80

An Eskimo child from the village of Noorvik, Alaska, once told a visitor: "My grandmother told me that when she looks at the snow, she thinks of me. When I look at the snow, I think of her. If I looked at the snow and there was no one to think of, I would be blind and deaf. The snow would fall on me, but it wouldn't be snow for me."

— ROBERT COLES

My own history, medically speaking, involved a mystery.

— Thomas De Quincey

CONTENTS

PART ONE

Slouching Towards Codeine

On November 15, 1972 — one week after Richard Nixon was reelected — I clapped my hands for fourteen hours and thirty-one minutes. I was listed in The Guinness Book of World Records. *I was eleven years old.*

My record was published on page 449 of the 1974 edition of the Guinness Book, *landlocked between the listings "Largest Circus" and "Club-Swinging," in the chapter entitled "Human Achievements":*

Clapping. The duration record for continuous clapping is 14 hours 31 minutes by Thomas C. Andrews (b. April 30, 1961) at Charleston, West Virginia, on November 15, 1972. He sustained an average of 120 claps per minute and an audibility range of at least 100 yards.

SKATING ON ONE GALOSH

He was a great walker. Oh! An astonishing
walker . . .
—Constantin Righas on Rimbaud in Ethiopia

I have traveled a good deal in Ann Arbor.
But not this morning. You wouldn't think I'd been walk-
ing upright for very long if you watched me step from the
University of Michigan bus this morning. I stepped onto a
pockmarked pool of ice on the sidewalk at Fletcher Street.
The ice hissed and ached under my feet.

My feet — first the right foot, then both together — skidded
for a second before sliding out from under me. For that one
second, maybe less, I was an astonishing walker, skating
across the ice before finding myself airborne, pewter trees and
yew bushes flashing by. I remember fretting over the where-
abouts of the library book I was carrying — Walter Savage
Landor's *Imaginary Conversations* — and the letter I'd placed
inside it. The letter was from William Stafford, a poet I admire extravagantly and whose letters I cherish. Then I landed
on my right leg and my back, heard a sound like that of a fist
flattening a tomato, and felt my ankle grind and twist in its
socket. I should have been thinking, *Factor VIII, factor VIII,*
factor VIII . . .

But I did not think of factor VIII (the blood-clotting agent
that I, as a "classical" hemophiliac, lack). It's strange what
rushes through the mind during trauma. Lying on my back on
the slickened sidewalk, in the beginning moments of a serious

bleed, I thought about the time years ago when I held a knife to my brother's throat.

———————

The image often haunts and inhabits me when I begin a bleed.

John and I were in the upstairs hallway of our house in the suburbs of Charleston, West Virginia. It must have been 1973. John was in high school; I was just starting junior high.

I'd been looking around the neighborhood. The Rafferty brothers shot BB guns at each other. They threw lit matches and firecrackers, too. Mike Scheller pushed his brother Max off their backyard tree house, breaking Max's arm. Bob Lilley tried to outline his sister Claire's torso with darts against the Raffertys' garage door. A dart nicked her thigh. I was scared to death of the violence of these "pranks." Such pranks were ubiquitous, though, among the kids in our neighborhood. Nothing comparable ever happened between John and me. Were we abnormal? Worse, were we sissies? Clearly something was missing. Danger. How to infuse it?

John had just come out of the bathroom, squinting at the light from a ceiling fixture hanging above the bathroom door. Light dazzled and appalled John. His eyes, which kidney disease had made apractic and unreliable, never got used to light's glare and shimmer. He would sit for hours in darkness on the edge of his bed, utterly at ease.

No doubt, I had seen a move like this on TV — on *The Mod Squad,* say, or *The Streets of San Francisco.* My plan was to scare him and wait for his retaliation. I'd scare him, he'd scare me, our lives would be richer. Of course, I knew that as a dialysis patient, he was pathetically vulnerable. He possessed an utter lack of coordination, his vision dimmed periodically, his growth was stunted to four foot eleven, he moved through the world at a snail's pace. I had never taken advantage of his vulnerability. It was uncharacteristic of me, to say the least. My role, I'd decided long before, was to protect John to the best of my ability, to be, if not his keeper, then at least his callow bodyguard. But on this day I decided we needed to spice up our moldering lives with a little danger, fear, and artifice. We could never compete with the Raffertys, but we could pretend for a while that we had Rafferty-like vacuity.

I held John's old pocketknife in my hand, its blunt blade tucked away.

"Ever been held up?" I said, opening the knife. I tried to sound tough and vacuous. The blade was short and scarred.

"Nope," John said. He looked distractedly at the knife in my hand. He was supremely uninterested.

"What would happen if I held you up—like this?" I held the knife to his throat. It felt awkward, and silly. John and I hadn't so much as wrestled in years.

I wasn't serious. John knew that. But I said nothing. John didn't seem surprised. He simply said, matter-of-factly, "Great. You're pulling a knife on me."

Immediately his body relaxed. It slumped into submission. *You're stronger, I won't fight you,* his body said. I was confused. After all, I was twelve. John was seventeen. *My* body was weak. His abdication of what I saw as his responsibility to fight back, to defy me, his acceptance of my so-called strength, startled and saddened me.

I withdrew the knife.

For the first time I realized the extent to which John had accepted his disease.

To my twelve-year-old mind, acceptance of disease, of extreme vulnerability, was anathema. One had to defy one's illness with all the energy one could summon. Defiance was crucial to survival. For a long time I thought John shared this view. As children, we were like all the other kids we knew: out of the sight of parents, we tried to behave as shockingly as we knew how. We drew the line at physical cruelty to each other. Neither of us had a knack for it, try as we might. Still, worldliness was a style we wore; no, it was the hidden and authentic double to our inauthentic, polite, churchgoing selves. John's acceptance — of his disease, his doctors, his parents — represented to me a giving in to the forces of darkness.

There was something else, too. John not only accepted his illness but appeared grateful for it. I'd heard his prayers. He thanked God for kidney disease. I was baffled, but I was also listening.

John was an inscrutable and constant presence in my life. Since his death in 1980, his presence has only intensified. Memory tends to purify and ossify the images of loved ones; I want to fight against that impulse absolutely, especially as I remember John.

John had at least one major operation each year for the last seven years of his life. He underwent, among other procedures, two total hip replacements, a kidney transplant (for which he had been on a waiting list for years), an operation to remove the transplanted kidney (after it failed along with his ruined spleen), and an operation to remove his gallbladder (which happened to follow a horrifying battle with pancreatitis).

Except for the three years he had the transplant, he required dialysis every other day from the time he was sixteen. In 1979, after the operation to remove his spleen and transplanted kidney, my mother and father were told that an artery had accidentally been clipped during the procedure, with the result that John's system retained fluids. Toxins pooled in his cells; the cells sputtered and drowned in poison. It was the beginning of the end. He died the following spring.

To the extent that our mutual illnesses allowed, we tormented each other constantly. We plotted intricate revenge on those who wrought humiliations at school. John was never able to go outside to play. Thus, our play usually consisted of housebound intellectual terrorism. We dissected each other's friends and favorite books and movies and TV shows as if they were floating in a pool of formaldehyde. We listened to Led Zeppelin and a hundred other bands and argued fiercely about their places in the rock music canon. To be stupid was to be invisible, or dead. John was smart — about people, about music. His high school buddies called him Mini-Brute. The name averred that although kidney disease stunted his growth to four foot eleven, he was one of the guys. He was *bad*.

Then, sometime during his junior year in high school, he became a saint.

His transformation was more gradual than the last sentence suggests, but to me it was like watching a movie in fastforward. One minute he is listening with manic glee to Jimi Hendrix, the next he is burning his record albums because they are a hindrance to God's plan for us. One minute he is brilliantly savaging Dean Martin's appearance on *The Tonight Show*, the next he is saying only good things about people.

I have in my life occasionally flirted with piety. John married it. He became one of those whom Saint Augustine in the

Confessions called the *servi Dei,* the servants of God, pious men and women whose faith remains unshaken by the cruelest circumstances. He decided to become baptized again, this time as an adult, to correspond to the adult evolution of his will. He and my parents became partners in an Amway business — AAA [Andrews, Andrews and Andrews] & Associates, their business card read. Amway made up a kind of subculture within evangelical circles in West Virginia. Fellow Amway dealers often came to our house to pray with John, to touch him, to have him pray *for* them. He would sit in his dialysis chair, a green La-Z-Boy recliner facing the TV in the "green room," the family room, and receive visitors as though they were suppliants. From upstairs or down the hall I heard the voices. I heard normal conversations that at some point took on a sudden, strange hush as John and his visitors began praying, speaking in tongues, laying hands on one another.

As they left the house, I studied the faces of those Amway dealers. They appeared changed, transformed for a while by hope or courage. One woman stopped me as I rode my bicycle on the driveway, placing her hands firmly, even brutally, on the handlebars.

"You know your brother's a saint," she said. "God put him here to be a witness to His glory. You might want to pay attention before it's too late."

Before it's too late. Too late for John? Did she think John was going to die soon? No. She clearly meant *me,* before it's too late for me. I might die unsaved and live forever in hellfire. From which fate John could apparently play a mediatory role in delivering me.

Had John's transformation from disease-challenged suburban kid to saint exacted any toll? Did he miss the easy confidence we shared, the endless discussions of pop culture, the genuine affection of his peers? We had had the brotherhood of pain and illness to unite us, a bond I thought as undying as actual brotherhood. The boundaries that illness created — though I fought against them while John seemed at home nowhere else — were themselves an irreducible connection. Suddenly all that had changed. His canonization took him away from me before his death. Now I realize that his religious fervor increased exactly as his health diminished. He knew he was going to die — if not during an upcoming operation, then not long afterward. He was making preparations. He was practicing for death. He became very good at it.

And now here I was years later, splayed across the Fletcher Street sidewalk, experiencing the kind of vulnerability that John knew so well.

I looked around me. Behind me was the Rackham Building, a huge, deliciously gloomy structure housing the Michigan Society of Fellows and the offices of, among others, the *Michigan Quarterly Review*. Across the street from the bus stop, the morning sun glared off the glass front of the Power Center, a performing-arts space where recently I'd attended a lecture by the architect Michael Graves. The lecture was on the "postmodern object." Now I felt like a postmodern object myself: dissembling, unsure of its status, suffused with crisis.

My breath plumed and disappeared.

The surprise of the event paralyzed me for a moment. I felt as though the synapses in my brain were misfiring, emptying me of speech or motor skills. Dimly I noticed figures stepping with exaggerated weariness across the icy sidewalk. One drew near to me. It was a tall, round, large-necked undergraduate. Or so I thought. He was holding an oversized textbook of some kind in his left hand. Blond and deeply tanned, he wore a blue baseball cap and a blue University of Michigan sweatshirt. And he was wearing shorts — baggy brown shorts in the middle of winter. The jarring incongruity of his shorts and the temperature — thirty-four degrees, I'd heard on the radio before leaving the apartment — brought me, as it were, to my senses.

"Okay, man?" asked this improbable and radiant angel of mercy.

"Um," I said.

"You probably sprained it," he said as he helped me up off the sidewalk. "You'll be fine."

Suddenly I was upright. My head was spinning. Baggy Shorts was walking away. Then he turned back and said, "Don't take your shoe off."

"What's that?" I said, still dizzy. I was in the way of people trying to get on and off the bus. I hopped out of the way as best I could.

"Your shoe. Don't take it off. As soon as you take it off, it'll swell like a mother."

"Good idea. Thanks for your help."

"No problem," he said. And then he said something that at first unnerved and then delighted me: "I'm a doctor."

Had I heard him? "You mean you're in medical school?" I asked, thinking I was being generous by taking his remark seriously.

"No. I'm a doctor," he said. He smiled wearily, as if he had to convince people of his profession every day. His broad tan face was enormously engaging.

Baggy Shorts walked off. This time he did not look back.

Was he a doctor? No, he was obviously too young. Still, he declared his vocation so nonchalantly, even self-deprecatingly, but at the same time with such authority that I had to wonder. In no way did he betray himself as a joker or poser. But no, no, it was ridiculous. He looked like one of my students. He looked *younger* than many of my students. And what would a doctor be doing wearing shorts in the middle of winter? Then again, was I so committed to appearances that I thought all doctors had to have a certain look? If he wasn't a doctor, then I loved the fact that he saw me as gullible, that he thought he could make such an outrageous statement and walk out of my life. If he *was* a doctor, then I loved the fact that he wore shorts in the middle of winter and looked like an undergraduate: what teasing he must endure from his colleagues!

———

I could tell that blood was pumping into my right ankle and calf and possibly into the right knee as well. I knew I had to get an infusion. The pain was not great—no worse than a badly sprained ankle. The serious pain would come later. It was biding its time. But there is a sensation—which took me years to identify and trust—that tells me I have started a bleed. It is a tingling inside the joint, a persistent thin kiss prolonged to the point of discomfort. The discomfort grows and grows until enough blood has filled the joint to press against the nerve endings.

Now I felt that slight unmistakable kiss.

I sat down. I cupped my hands under my leg and held it up in the air, keeping the knee joint as straight as possible. Blood would soon try to bend the joint, to find more room to bleed into.

With Baggy Shorts gone, I had to figure out how to get to the emergency room. Why didn't I think to ask him for a ride? Did the fact that he didn't offer one mean he wasn't a doctor after all?

The University of Michigan Hospital is not far from Fletcher Street. In fact, the bus I had just so unastonishingly departed stopped at the corner of Catherine Street and Fuller Avenue, near a back entrance to the hospital. I wouldn't have to walk as far, though, if I took the bus all the way back to my apartment on McIntyre Avenue. My wife, Carrie, would be home, working on the computer graphics course she taught in the art department. She'd take me to the emergency room. From the apartment I could call my bosses. I was working as a copyeditor for *Mathematical Reviews* (MR) and as an adjunct lecturer in creative writing at the University of Michigan. The collisions between mathematics and poetry were often startling. On Monday, Wednesday, and Friday afternoons I would stop editing papers with titles like "Asymptotic Behavior of the Probability of Error of the Likelihood Ratio Test in the Discrimination of Point Processes with Continuous Compensators," leave the *MR* office on Fourth Street, then walk up William Street to Angell Hall, where my class would discuss poems such as Wallace Stevens's "Not Ideas about the Thing but the Thing Itself." I needed to call both employers to let them know what had happened to me.

I waited for the bus. I thought of a line of Kafka's: "I wait like an ox." A good line, I thought, but now that my waiting carried some authority, some urgency, does it stand up? The line assumed that oxen wait patiently, exemplarily. Do they? How would Kafka know, sitting in his Prague apartment with a view of a brick wall? How would anyone who wasn't an ox know? He might as well have said, "I wait like a cow." Not true. The thick, quick bluntness of *ox* (*Ochse* in the original German), its heaviness on the tongue, its surprising power when conjoined with the suddenly meager pronoun I *(ich)*, made it absolutely the right word. *I wait like an ox*. Yes.

Why was I thinking about that?

It's strange what rushes through the mind during trauma. The mind delays or interrupts or doles out as if in pieces the inevitable confrontation with the facts of a traumatic event. This happens in hundreds of ways. For me, it usually involves thinking of John or an obsessive fascination with language. Again and again I've watched my mind deliver a troublesome or felicitous image of John or a troublesome or felicitous sentence to the forefront of consciousness during bleeds, like a thief who says, "Look, your shoe's untied!" before swiping your purse. Not that these images and sentences arrive uninvited. I welcome them. At some point I recognized that my mind during bleeds would not sit still, would misbehave, would jump unpredictably from image to image, thought to thought, delivering strangeness, irrelevance, irreverence. For years I fought against it. I thought it meant I was weak-willed. Eventually I learned to relax and let my mind leap and turn as eccentrically as it needed.

People were milling about, trying not to look at me sitting on the sidewalk holding my leg up. I glanced at *Imaginary Conversations,* made sure William Stafford's letter was safe inside it. As I waited, as blood rushed into my calf and ankle, I became flooded with a sense of sheer, impersonal luck.

———

Let me explain.

It was the middle of January 1989. Six years earlier, in September 1982, Dr. Bruce Evatt at the Centers for Disease Control (CDC) suggested that factor VIII concentrate transmitted HIV, the AIDS virus. When my hematologist told me to assume that I had HIV even if I tested negative, I wrote in a notebook:

> *The words* HIV *and* AIDS. *Even overheard by chance — especially overheard by chance — they provoke psychological tremors that I associate with the*

Hebrew idea of the Tetragrammaton: unfathomable
depths informing the slightest twinge or shimmer of
consciousness.

Between 1982 and 1985, when the first test to screen do-
nated blood became available, each bleed posed a macabre
dilemma. Should I treat it aggressively with factor VIII and
risk HIV, or should I let the bleed run its course and risk permanent crippling or even death by prolonged hemorrhaging?

My hematologists always sided with factor VIII. Inclined to
relieve pain and fend off long-term disability, they down-
played the risk of infection. They made a distinction — reasonable enough, on the surface — between a real threat and a
potential threat. "Treat the real threat now," my hematologists said. "Worry about the potential threat later." I con-
curred.

Hematologists continued to recommend factor VIII concentrate for a simple reason. It represented a miracle. Introduced
in the early 1970s, factor VIII transformed a generation of hemophiliacs from dependents of the health-care system to fully
engaged citizens. For the first time, hemophiliacs could infuse
themselves at home or at work. Unemployment among hemophiliacs plummeted, as did the average number of work-
days hemophiliacs lost each year to bleeds. The world had apparently opened itself up to hemophiliacs at last, thanks to
factor VIII. Hematologists were very reluctant to advise patients to stop using it.

In my case, the argument for treatment was compelling, to
say the least: the complications that can result from untreated
bleeds require *more* factor VIII than does the original bleed.
And yet the numbers are staggering: some 90 percent of hemophiliacs who had repeated infusions between 1978 and
early 1985 carry HIV.

I'd had repeated infusions between 1978 and early 1985. So when my hematologist told me to assume I had HIV even if I tested negative, I thought she was simply being realistic. One hemophiliac after another tested positive. In fact, every adult hemophiliac I'd ever met was infected.

That's when it struck me: *Carrie*. Had I infected her? We'd always used condoms, except for a brief interval when she was on the Pill. Had I dragged Carrie — *Carrie!* — down with me into the pit of terror and fear and unknowing that was HIV and AIDS?

Then again, what if I was infected and she was not? What would happen to our sex life? Would we trust condoms? We'd discussed it; we both wanted to be 100 percent certain that Carrie would not be infected. Even 99 percent certainty was unacceptable. What would make us feel safe — two condoms? Two condoms and withdrawal before ejaculation? There were, of course, other ways to express ourselves sexually, but would we forgo altogether the richness and voluptuousness and mutual engulfment of intercourse?

We tried our best not to panic. We decided to wait and see if I developed any symptoms before confronting the specter of this pandemic by taking the test. In the meantime we would use condoms and nonoxynol-9, which contains substances that destroy HIV.

Friends, including doctors, gave us conflicting advice. Some said we needed to know my HIV status for our peace of mind. Not knowing, they said, would torment us more than a positive test result would. "Let's say you do test positive," my old philosophy professor said to me. "You won't be hiding your head in the sand. To me, that would be the important thing. I mean, don't you want to *know*, once and for all?"

"Sure I do," I said. "Then again, there's that great line of Beckett's. 'Who knows what the ostrich sees in the sand?'"

"That's easy," the philosopher said. "It sees sand."

Others suggested that as long as I was *not* tested, I could always say — on a job application or on a request for medical insurance — that I had never tested positive for HIV. The benefits of not knowing, in terms of work and insurance coverage, outweighed the assurance of knowing. Surprisingly, this was the view held by most of my friends who were doctors. They'd seen too many cases of discrimination, institutional and social. And, they said, in the absence of an effective course of treatment against AIDS, no one really knew what to do with the information of a positive test result.

Anytime I had a sinus infection, or white spots or sores inside my mouth, or diarrhea, or lumps in my neck or underarms, or persistent fatigue, or skin rashes, I was sure I was becoming symptomatic. But still I did not get tested, for fear that the test result would not remain confidential. In the air were horror stories of infected hemophiliacs who had lost their jobs, been dropped by their insurance companies, been told to leave their school districts. Outraged and pusillanimous neighbors even burned down one Florida family's house.

In 1987 Carrie and I moved to Ann Arbor, where the test was readily available through the hemophilia clinic at the University of Michigan Hospital. By that time the staff at the clinic was used to dealing with issues of discrimination. Sheryl Phillips, the hemophilia nurse coordinator at the clinic, assured me that the confidentiality of the test would be inviolable. After years of not knowing, Carrie and I were ready.

I tested negative.

I did not believe it. The odds were too much in favor of HIV. *I must be in the incubation period,* I thought, or *I've slipped into the small percentage of false negative test results.*

Carrie and I kept taking precautions. But after being tested at least once a year for the next few years, and testing negative each time, I finally came to trust the result. Then came what Carrie and I called the D-Day test. Instead of simply calling me up as she had done after my previous tests, Sheryl wrote me a letter:

Dear Tom —

Please call Lorna Baker or myself so we can make an appointment to talk with you.

Sheryl Phillips

Enclosed with the letter was the business card of Lorna Baker, a social worker who worked with the hemophilia clinic. Reading the letter, and seeing the social worker's card drop out unexpectedly, I thought: *Is this it? Is this how they contact you if you're HIV-positive, as opposed to the confident informality of the phone call made to those who tested negative? Was the hematologist who told me to assume that I carried HIV right after all? Why else would the social worker be involved?*

I called Sheryl and made an appointment.

When I showed up at the hemophilia clinic, Sheryl led me to a conference room, where I was to wait for the social worker. Sheryl said, "I'll go tell Lorna you're here," and left the room.

I thought: *That's it. There's no other way to read Sheryl's behavior. I tested positive. How should I break it to Carrie?*

"Fate, when not smiling on you, may be laughing at you." That line ran through my mind as I waited for Sheryl and the social worker to tell me the grim news. It had taken me a long time to trust my negative test results. Now that I was convinced I did not carry HIV, I tested positive. Fate was not only laughing at me, it was in hysterics.

A few minutes later Sheryl and the social worker entered the room together. Sheryl introduced me to Lorna Baker; we shook hands. They both sat down—gravely, I thought—across the table from me. "We want to talk to you about the results of your test."

I swallowed. "Yes," I said.

Sheryl looked at me. "Let me tell you right at the start that your test came out negative."

"!"

"What was that? Tom?"

"Um, nothing. Sorry."

Confused, relieved, drained, I gathered my wits enough to point out that the new method of getting in touch with me was a good way to stimulate and observe spontaneous ulcers, if not spontaneous combustion.

My HIV-negative status continued to baffle me. I was like my friend Steve, a gay man with, as he puts it, "a high-risk past." Steve tested negative for HIV while many of his friends, whose pasts were neither more nor less full of risk than his, tested positive.

"I feel out of the loop somehow," Steve told me during one of our long talks over beers at the Old Town, a bar in Ann Arbor. "I know that's crazy. But it's like, why am I so lucky? Sometimes when I get depressed, I wish I had HIV. At least then I'd have a reason to be depressed, a reason people could understand. And I'd be part of my community again. Is that sick or what?"

HIV-negative hemophiliacs play a different role in the hemophilia community than do HIV-negative gay men in the gay community. I am not surrounded by hemophiliacs, as Steve is by other gay men. None of my closest friends are hemophiliacs.

If I desired, I could ignore or avoid the HIV/AIDS tragedy in ways that would be impossible for a gay man.

But there are similarities. Both hemophiliacs and gay men have had HIV/AIDS thrust upon them as their central identifying characteristic within the culture at large. Both have had HIV/AIDS thrust upon them in more literal ways, too: insurance companies, for example, are obscenely effective in assigning hemophiliacs and gay men a common identity regardless of a particular individual's HIV/AIDS status.

Discussions about and within the hemophilia and gay communities turn almost invariably to HIV and AIDS. This is as it should be, of course. Nothing is more pressing or crucial to either community. And yet one must be able to raise other issues (the morality of genetic engineering, new orthopedic management techniques, the safety of prophylaxis for hemophiliac children, and so on) without feeling that one has committed the crime Bertolt Brecht invoked in his poem "To Those Born After":

> What times are these, when
> To speak about trees is almost a crime
> Because it implies silence about so many horrors?

At hemophilia conferences or gatherings, which are now rightly devoted to HIV and AIDS, HIV-negative hemophiliacs are like conscientious objectors admitted to a veterans hospital, though no conscientiousness is involved, no objection made.

There is no reason I do not carry HIV, just as there is no reason others do. I do not believe, that is, that God parcels out disease and agonizing death, deciding who receives them and who does not on the basis of moral or spiritual capabilities or shortcomings. Disease is a fact—simple, brutal, un-yielding—and it is a fact shot through with chance. Statistically, I should carry HIV. I do not. I do not, and while I want to avoid being sentimental, I can't deny my relief.

Chance had given me hemophilia. Now it appeared that chance had brought about the conditions whereby I avoided HIV and AIDS. How? Why? AIDS, like hemophilia, is a question without an answer. Or the answer is Antonin Artaud's, who said, "Chance is myself."

———

Though techniques for purifying factor VIII were made available in early 1985, no one would say with certainty that the blood supply was absolutely safe. Between 1982 and early 1985—between the CDC's report of AIDS among hemophiliacs and the availability of purified factor VIII concentrate—hemophiliacs had little reason to trust their well-intended and optimistic hematologists.

I remember the first time I saw AIDS introduced as a topic of concern among the hemophilia community in Michigan. It was in the November 1982 issue of *The Artery* (word of honor, that's the title), the newsletter of the Hemophilia Foundation of Michigan. The cover story was in the format of answers to frequently asked questions about the new and baffling disease. The document is remarkable largely for its self-contradictions. Early on in the story is the following exchange:

QUESTION: What are the causes?
ANSWER: The cause of AIDS is unknown. There are several theories, but none have been proven. The most widely known theory presently is that it is caused by a virus that attacks the immune cell.
QUESTION: How does one get it?

ANSWER: This, too, is unknown since the cause is unknown. However, the most widely held theory is that if the cause is a virus, it can be transmitted to individuals in a manner similar to the hepatitis B virus. That is, by contact with blood or blood products. . . .

Later, on the same page:

QUESTION: Should the hemophiliac change or stop his treatment with factor VIII or factor IX?

ANSWER: At the present time there is no specific evidence to warrant changing the use of factor VIII or factor IX.

The cautious among us developed a suspicious cast of mind that has been difficult to shed. A kind of wartime-rationing mentality set in, even after purified factor VIII concentrate became available: if at all possible, take the punishment and absorb the bleed. In January 1986 came the first CDC report of a patient infected with HIV as a result of a transfusion of *tested* blood. (At that time the test was known to be sensitive 95 percent of the time, leaving a window of error of 5 percent.) As late as 1987, when asked point-blank about the safety of the blood supply, all my hematologist could say was "We think it's very safe now."

To my ear, the word *think* in that sentence was fumigated by italics.

In 1989 the blood supply was safe. I knew it intellectually. The chances of contracting HIV from factor VIII were about one in forty thousand. As a hemophiliac who had raced motorcycles, this was a risk I could accept. But still, it was hard not to suspect misinformation, hard to trust blood companies and hematologists after six years of confusing and contradictory messages.

Today, though, as I sat on the sidewalk holding up my leg, I knew that there would be no risk at all. Today I would be infused with desmopressin acetate (DDAVP), a synthetic blood-clotting agent not derived from plasma. DDAVP had just been made available to me; I'd used it about three months ago when I broke and bled into my left ankle after a basketball accident. DDAVP stimulates what little active factor VIII my blood-stream carries and increases it to about 35 percent of normal. Thirty-five percent is adequate to treat "bleeds of a non-life-threatening nature," as the letter I carry in my wallet puts it. As a synthetic agent, DDAVP carries no risk of infection. Infusing it gives me a fever and chills, but it is worth every shiver.

My bus came. I clenched Landor's *Imaginary Conversations* as tightly as I could, afraid it would slip as I negotiated the steps and aisle. Hoisting myself by the railing inside the bus and then sort of hopping and swinging down the aisle, I found two empty seats together and sat down across them, propping up my leg. A young woman and a child, both bundled up in scarves and down coats, sat across the aisle from me. I opened *Imaginary Conversations* to the page where William Stafford's letter rested. The book opened to a dialogue between Sir Isaac Newton and Newton's teacher, the mathematician and theologian Isaac Barrow. Landor imagined the conversation to take place in 1668, on the day before Newton received his master's degree.

NEWTON: Sir, in a word, ought a studious man to think of matrimony?

BARROW: Painters, poets, mathematicians, never ought: other studious men, after reflecting for twenty years upon it, may. Had I a son of your age, I would not leave him in a grazing country. Many a man has been safe among cornfields, who falls a victim on the grass under an elm. There are lightnings very fatal in such places.

NEWTON: Supposing me no mathematician, I must reflect then for twenty years!

BARROW: Begin to reflect on it after twenty; and continue to reflect on it all the remainder: I mean at intervals, and quite leisurely.

I closed the book. The pain was starting to command attention. Isaac Barrow's views (or rather Landor's view of Barrow's views) of the deleterious effect of marriage were not what I needed just then, not when I was starting a bleed, which always added intense stress to my relationship with Carrie. Besides, Landor's Barrow was patronizing. The effects of marriage, in my experience, were anything but deleterious. Carrie and I had discovered a closeness and ease with each other I didn't know were possible before we married. *Yes, "there are lightnings very fatal in such places,"* I thought, admiring the balance and heft of that line, but they are mercifully fatal — fatal to one's frightened, insular self. Anyway, I was bringing the book to *Mathematical Reviews* to show Walter. Walter was one of *MR*'s luminous and charmingly deranged editors and a confirmed (as they say) bachelor. He would get a kick out of Landor.

I took William Stafford's letter out of its envelope. I wanted to hear Bill's curiosity, his calm and easy intimacy with the world, before pain made reading out of the question.

6 Jan 89

Headlong at my chores out here, I pause to think of the scene where you are—snow, I suspect. Out here it is overcast but mild, and I might even have to mow my lawn again before spring. We go up the mountains for our winter; there is plenty there, with snow as high as the car when we cross Santiam Pass.

Please learn all the lore thereabouts for when we next have a chance to meet; I'll do my part in my meanderings, the next notable one being around Massachusetts in February.

It was no use; reading was impossible. Serious, artless pain was coming on like a thunderstorm a hundred miles down the road and headed my way, flashing and roaring on the horizon. No matter. Let it come. *Let it come,* I thought. I was having a "non-life-threatening" bleed. I would see Carrie. I would receive an infusion of DDAVP. Someone would bring me codeine. Eventually I would be fine. "The sin against the Holy Ghost is ingratitude," the English poet Christopher Smart tells us. If so, then for once I was on good terms with that mysterious intercessor.

"*Does he have to do that?*" *the waitress at Pizza Hut asked. She passed out glasses of ice water from a tray, then set the tray down on the table.*

"*He's breaking a world record,*" *John said flatly.*

"*Does it bother you?*" *my mother said.* "*I can't make him stop, but we can leave.*"

The waitress looked up. "*You're joking, right? Let me see.*" *She gestured for me to pull my hands out from under the table.*

I showed my hands. Eyes, hostile, were staring from neighboring booths and tables.

"*He has to sustain an audibility range of at least a hundred yards,*" *John said.*

"*I'm getting the cook,*" *she said.* "*He's got to see this.*"

A minute later a thin man with botched teeth, wearing a blue dough-smeared apron, was glaring at me. "*Well,*" *he said impatiently,* "*let's see your deal.*"

Again I showed my hands. I speeded up, just a little, the rate of clapping.

"*Right. Unbelievable,*" *the cook said, shaking his head and disappearing.*

I said, "*Can we order?*"

"*What do you do if you have to go to the bathroom?*" *the waitress asked.*

"*I'd like a root beer,*" *I said.* "*Do you have root beer?*"

"He's trying to go the whole day without going," my mother said.

"Good luck!" the waitress said.

I said, "Do you have root beer?"

"Yeah, they have root beer," John said.

I said, "I was asking her, thank you very much."

"I don't think I could go the whole day," the waitress said. "I think I have a weak bladder."

I leaned over to John and whispered: "Help."

"Hey," said the waitress, "how are you going to eat pizza?"

"I'm not," I said. "I'm just sipping some root beer. If you have it."

"They have it, they have it," John said, and buried his head in his hands.

"I'm going to feed him," my mother said.

"No way!" I said.

For a second I forgot to clap, then caught myself and reestablished my rhythm.

"We'll have a large mushroom and pepperoni," my mother said. "And I'd like a glass of iced tea. What do you want to drink?"

"I want a Coke," John said.

"Root beer," I said.

THE PROFESSIONAL HEMOPHILIAC
AND THE ELVIS QUIZ

They are usually well between attacks of bleeding.
— ROY R. KRACKE, *Diseases of the Blood* (1941)

THE PROFESSIONAL HEMOPHILIAC

Recently I heard a radio program about the songs of various North American birds. The white-throated sparrow, the program's host explained, sings two songs. The first song assures the wilderness within earshot: *I am a white-throated sparrow.* The second song announces something else entirely: *I am this particular white-throated sparrow.*

Writing this book, I can sing with assurance only that second song. To presume otherwise would be to set myself up as some kind of professional hemophiliac, recklessly confident that I speak for all bleeders. To a certain extent then, I disagree with the idea behind personal accounts of illness such as this one. To put it another way: this book, by its very nature, flirts with a way of thinking about illness that I believe is dangerous and seductive to the ill. The battle is over identity. Every day the question arises: Am I a hemophiliac who happens to be a writer (or cashier or househusband or whatever), or am I a writer who happens to be a hemophiliac?

I remember a pickup basketball game in Ann Arbor during which I momentarily lost this battle. I was playing with a group of college-age jocks whom I didn't know, and I stunk up the court. I couldn't have put the ball into the Grand Canyon. The pleasure of playing a hard game of basketball well, with no one's knowing or suspecting that I'm a hemophiliac (even though I am constantly assessing the court with an eye out for dangerous situations to avoid), is similar to the pleasure of being mistaken for a native while visiting a foreign country. On that day, though, I was the ugly American abroad in the country of basketball. I got furiouser and furiouser. When the game was over, I started over to the fellow who had played point guard on my team; he controlled the flow of the ball and made sure I didn't get within ten feet of it. He was walking toward a water fountain where his buddies were lining up to get a drink.

"What's the deal?" I said angrily. Surprised, he turned around to face me. I backed down, suddenly embarrassed. (What was I going to do, pick a fight? The scenario was absurd, like a bad movie — *Rambo XIII: The Hemophiliac's Revenge*.) I muttered, "Sorry. It's just that . . . never mind. Sorry." He turned back to his friends.

I was about to say, "It's just that I'm a hemophiliac." I shuddered: I'd just lost the battle, and I knew it.

Once a hemophiliac starts using hemophilia as an excuse, once he (hemophilia, with extremely rare exceptions, occurs only in males) allows himself the status of victim, then the word *survival* is leached of meaning. You may survive the disease, but it has defeated you.

Of course, periodic lapses such as the one I experienced at the basketball court are natural. It's important to give yourself a break when they occur, in order to learn from them rather than to deny them. But I am a "survivor" of hemophilia, as I say, only to the extent that I am able to move beyond such lapses, beyond victimization.

Why then write a book about hemophilia, if hemophilia is only one of the stories my life tells me, not *the* story?

To me there is a central justification for such a book: to de-mythologize illness, for myself and (one hopes but cannot presume) others, revealing it not as a rarified tragedy but as the commonplace event it is. Demythologizing illness requires the work of a great many people. A hemophiliac's role in this project, I believe, is to be absolutely candid about what happens to him during a typical bleed. By "bleed" I mean the following series of events. A blood vessel (or vessels) breaks, releasing blood into a joint and the surrounding muscles. Clotting factor is given in an IV drip to retard the bleeding, but it takes time for the infusion to take effect. Meanwhile, blood fills the joint. The pain is staggering. The limb locks. The muscles atrophy. One is faced with weeks of waiting for the body to absorb the blood, followed by weeks of physical therapy to straighten and regain the joint's original range of motion.

I want here to re-create one hemophiliac's response to an accident. I have not chosen an "ideal" bleed. That is, there is much about my reaction to the traumatized ankle and about my interaction with doctors that I am not proud of. "Warts and all or not at all" was my guiding principle. There is occasional pettiness, and childishness, on my part. There is spinelessness. There is misguided anger. Above all, there is the flurry of thought and fear, which eventually gives way to the surprising, implausible surge of convalescence, the spirit's if not the body's, a convergence of self and world that opens one's eyes to the mysterious in the familiar after a season in hell.

———

But I'm getting ahead of myself.

———

THE ELVIS QUIZ

The bus smelled of tuna fish. Someone behind me was eating a sandwich.

Conversations that lulled as I hopped and swung to my seat now resumed. Eavesdropping is an occupational hazard of writers. But my desire to listen to the various conversations on the bus, to hear each voice's nuance and vibrancy, was more ferocious than the impulse to eavesdrop on any particular one. It was a way to remind myself that the world goes about its business, inexhaustible, unforeseeable, with comforting disregard of me and my bleeding. That may sound morose. It is not. Letting sense impressions sink into me, as into a fossil bed, with bright particularity confirms the otherness and blessed solidity of the world's presence. The smell of tuna fish, for instance. The black rubber mat running along the floor of the bus. The cowboy hat on the head of the man in front of me. That the world is present, and that its presence is not a comment on my hemophilia, is a lesson I can't be reminded of too often when I am undergoing a bleed. The temptation is to turn so inward that the world exists only as a billboard of my fear and pain.

My perforated and throbbing leg draped across the bus seat, the pain building momentum toward its noxious pitch, I was desperate to turn outward. I listened in to a middle-aged man in the front row. A tattered backpack was slung over his shoulder. He was lecturing the bus driver, practically shouting over the bus's pneumatic gasps and lurches:

"Kellogg's is the most beautiful plant anywhere. Beautiful company. White hats, white hats there. I'd eat a flake off their floor. I don't eat things off floors."

"That right?" said the bus driver.

"Battle Creek. You know it. Beautiful plant. Beautiful. White hats, I tell you."

"Uh-huh," said the bus driver.

White hats, white hats there.

The world going about its business. Yes.

I tuned in to the conversation directly behind me. It was between two young women — undergraduates, I assumed — unless, of course, they were doctors.

One said, "Is *trash can* one word or two?"

"Two," the other said authoritatively.

"Shit!" cried the first. "I missed that one!"

I tried to imagine the quiz on which one would find the question: *Which is correct* — trash can *or* trashcan? Nothing came to mind.

I looked at the young woman and child across the aisle from me. Were they hearing what I was hearing? They didn't appear to be listening, deep in exchanges of their own. Occasionally the child, a boy of two or three, would give me furtive sideways glances. I held my leg up when the bus bounced over a pothole in the road. I grimaced. When I did, the child would tug at the young woman's sleeve and point.

"Don't point," said the young woman.

———

The bus dragged on toward North Campus and Married Student Housing. The man with the backpack got off near the hospital.

"Have a good day now," the bus driver said to the man.

"You know I will. Take care of yourself."

"Planning on it," said the bus driver.

As soon as the doors closed on the man with the backpack, the bus driver looked in his mirror to find a woman near the front row. Obviously picking up a suspended conversation, he said, "Like I said, I missed *Falcon Crest* last week. You think Emma and R.D. are getting married tonight?"

"You know how it is with Emma," said the woman. "She'll find a way. If not tonight, then another night. She keeps me on my toes." She laughed, and the bus driver laughed with her.

Suddenly, outrageously, a familiar voice popped into my head, with a lewd and bizarre question:

"When can we finger you?"

———

This time I recognized instantly the chain of association. Hearing the conversation about *Falcon Crest* reminded me of Terry's brother. Terry was one of my supervisors at *Mathematical Reviews*. She had a brother who starred in the daytime soap opera *As the World Turns*. Terry updated us, the copyeditors at *MR,* daily on the show's progress in her computer finger.plan. A finger.plan was an on-line bulletin board where *MR* employees offered philosophical ramblings, traded recipes (a fellow who worked in the library put together a forty-page list of every type of rice available in the Midwest), or simply announced what had happened to them during the previous twenty-four hours ("Last night Cliff Jr., our four-year-old, learned a new phrase: *of course*. '*Of course,* I'm going to eat the cookies,' he says when you tell him not to. '*Of course,* I'm going outside to play.' Parenthood is bliss, let me tell you!").

My introduction to finger.plans occurred during my first day at *MR,* as I met the copyediting department for the first time.

I was all sincerity and nerves. Nancy, my chief supervisor, introduced me to the department, which consisted of twelve other copyeditors and the "Blond Translators." The Blond Translators were two women, Anne-Marie and Barbara, who between them translated all the reviews submitted in Romance and Germanic languages. On the wall were posters of grim-faced mathematicians: David Hilbert, Emmy Noether, Srinivasa Ramanujan, Hermann Weyl.

"We call this room the Wormhole," Nancy said. "And we call our department the Fuzzy Sets." Twelve Fuzzy Sets looked up at me from their respective desks. (The Blond Translators had their own office down the hall.)

"Ah," I said.

I found myself staring at Nancy's teeth, their pronounced overbite. The overbite was not a flaw. It gave her face definition, solidity.

Taped to Nancy's office door was an oversized letter, handwritten in crayon, to Santa Claus: *Dear Santa, I am allergic to sulfa drugs. Please don't bring me sulfa drugs.*

Just then Sharon, a Fuzzy Set stooped under her desk lamp's oval of light, spoke up, addressing everyone in the room. She winked at me conspiratorially, as if I'd worked at *MR* for years. "What's the deal with the new paint job? Here we are, one of only three journals in the world that review papers in every area of mathematics. Then why is it" — she slammed her fist on her desk, lampooning passion — "why is it that our building has to look like a Taco Bell?"

Mark, a copyeditor whose slight beard, I learned later, earned him the title of Fuzziest Fuzzy Set, replied, "Yeah. I hear we're putting in a drive-in window."

Terry, the supervisor whose brother was on the soaps, said, "I'll have a spin-glass theory and a two-body problem to go, please." Everyone laughed. I laughed.

No partitions segmented the Wormhole: it was an open area, bathed in white light, where the Fuzzy Sets sat at ancient gray desks and talked, argued, joked, insulted and quizzed one another, giggled, shrieked. I was doomed. How could anyone edit surreally difficult mathematical texts and be witty at the same time?

I looked into each fatigued, well-lit face. A large woman with red hair and thick glasses came up to me and said, matter-of-factly, "When can we finger you?"

"I'm sorry?"

"Finger.plans. On the computer. They're daily messages you write to the whole department. To read somebody's finger.plan, you finger* them. Follow me."

I looked at Nancy. "Go on," Nancy said. "Gwen will take good care of you. I'll catch up with you later."

I followed Gwen across the room to a table with a Wyse computer on it. Her steps elicited low thuds from the floor. At the table she turned to me, shook my hand, and said, "I'm Gwen, by the way. Pull up a seat."

She logged on the computer, typed "@finger_CKB," pressed the Return key and waited. "We're fingering Caryn," she said. "Her initials are CKB."

In a few seconds words appeared on the monitor screen:

```
@finger_CKB:

         The Elvis Quiz

Q. What was Elvis's most beautiful feature
   on his head?
A. Easy. His hair.
Q. Is it true that the vest Elvis wore in
   1953 and 1954 has a mustard stain on it
   that's not visible in most photographs?
A. Yes.
Q. Is it true that Elvis could see both the
   things above him in the air and below
```

---

*This is unlike the "finger" command used in, say, UNIX e-mail accounts, which refers to the ability of the sender of an e-mail message to determine whether or not that message has been received.

```
      him in the water at the same time when
      he swam?
   A. No, you are thinking of the whirligig
      beetle.
   Q. In what song did Elvis claim to be itch-
      ing like a man in a fuzzy tree?
   A. "Crying in the Chapel."
```

"Caryn's really into music," Gwen said. "A lot of us are. If you like folk music—you like folk music?"

I started to answer, but Gwen continued before I had a chance. "If you like folk music, Caryn knows the folk scene inside and out. Suzanne Vega once slept on the floor of her apartment."

"She did?" I said, duly impressed.

"Yeah. Caryn's like a manager, publicist or something. You know the poet Marvin Bell?"

"Personally?" I said.

"His son's a folk singer. Pretty good, too."

"I didn't know that," I said.

Gwen typed "@finger_WBW" and hit the Return key. "Let's see what Bill's up to today," she said.

CKB's finger.plan disappeared, WBW's flickering onto the screen in its place:

```
@finger_WBW:

Sign (poem, really) on a telephone pole on
the corner of First and Jefferson:

          I hope the S.O.B.
          who stole our plants
          rots in hell!
```

```
Otherwise, here are my weekend plans. Fri-
day: Work on feminist criticism project for
UMI Press. Saturday: Pee-wee, Mighty Mouse,
then more feminist criticism. Hope to find
out what phallologocentrism means. Sunday:
Read Oedipus, watch Psycho, take shower,
call MOM.
```

"Ugh," Gwen said. "Well, that's the lowdown on fin-ger.plans. We expect a new one at least once a week. We're pretty desperate for distractions around here."

"Ah," I said. I misread her last comment to mean the lesson was over. I started to stand up.

Gwen wasn't finished. "Up for one more?" she asked. It was a rhetorical question. I settled back into my chair. "Who should it be? Who will it be?" Her voice simulated sinister intent, as if she were selecting her next victim for vivisection. "Who will it be?" Her hands rinsed themselves ominously. Knowingly or not, she was doing a fine Lon Chancy.

"How about Terry," she said, typing "@finger_TSH." With a studious forefinger she pushed her glasses up on her nose, abandoning her Lon Chaney imitation. "Her brother used to be on *As the World Turns*," Gwen said. "He still is, but they just killed him off. I mean, they're about to kill him off. I think."

```
@finger_TSH:

My brother was now an out-of-work actor. He
had toiled for four years on As the World
Turns, playing Dr. Casey Peretti, a brash
young surgeon who fell for the boss's
daughter; got his heart broken; fell for
his landlady (a nurse, mother, and night-
```

club chanteuse); married her; rescued his grown stepson from foreign ne'er-do-wells holding him hostage off the coast of Greece; had his surgical career cut short after falling ill with Guillain-Barré syndrome; and overcame the depression and bitterness that gripped him in his paraplegia. His character had finally been killed off by succumbing to encephalitis.

He had finished taping his hospital deathbed scenes the previous week for broadcast three weeks later, and was set to spend three weeks out of New York before facing the specter of unemployment. While bicycling in Central Park, he fell, damaged his arm, and landed in the hospital some days later with a raging case of septicemia. And what do you do when you're doped up, bored out of your skull, stuck in bed with your arm elevated and three IVs dripping into you? You watch the soaps. So there he was, lying in his hospital bed, watching himself lying in his hospital bed on TV. His doctor entered the room, did the requisite double take between patient-in-bed and patient-in-bed-on-TV, and remarked, "I must tell my colleagues about this."

"Whoa!" Gwen said exultantly. "That's awesome! I wish *I* had a brother on the soaps."

"Me, too," I said. And again, under my breath, "Me, too."

———

We hit a large pothole. The bus rattled. I gripped *Imaginary Conversations*. Pain stormed through my leg. My ability to pay attention, to translate sense-data into any kind of meaning, waned.

I looked at my right leg. I was alarmed but not surprised to see that under my sock a tennis ball had apparently affixed itself to the anklebone. I wanted to turn down my sock and have a look. *No,* I thought, *better to hold off till you get home. No need to alarm the little boy or risk scraping the skin against the chair as we hit another pothole. There's nothing I can do now anyway.*

The bus made its way down Fuller Avenue.

I wish I had a brother on the soaps. I tried to distract myself from my leg, to let my mind skate over my body like a water strider over the thin surface of a creek.

I tried to remember conversations John and I had had about TV shows, movies, music. I remembered John laughing, with a combination of disgust and camp pleasure, at my celebrations of *All in the Family,* Dick Cavett, *Monty Python and the Holy Grail,* the Ramones. But my thoughts veered obsessively to the knife episode. I couldn't help it. Again I heard John's voice:

Great. You're pulling a knife on me.

I had not replied to his utter resignation. Or had I misread him? What if I'd prodded him? How would he have responded?

Great. You're pulling a knife on me.

Of course I don't mean it. I'm joking. You know that, right?

Yeah, right. With a knife to my throat, I'll agree to anything.

You think I'd stab you?

Give me the knife. Then we'll talk.

There. Sorry.

Gotcha. You're so gullible!

Try again.

Great. You're pulling a knife on me.

Don't move.

This is just great.

Move and it's curtains.

Give me a break.

Move and it's curtain time.

That's my knife.

Do you confess?

That's my knife.

No, it isn't. Do you confess?

Confess to what?

I don't know. Think of something.

I confess to having the stupidest brother in the world. Who doesn't even know how to hold a knife.

Show me.

Try again.

Great. You're pulling a knife on me.

C'mon.

What?

C'mon.

What?

Take it away from me. You know, like on The Mod Squad.

No way, you dork.

C'mon.

No way.

Later?

No.

Never?

No.

No to never, *meaning yes sometime but not now, or* no *meaning never ever?*

No meaning never.

You used to fight.
When?
You used to beat me up all the time. When we were really little. Remember?
You must be thinking of your other brother with kidney disease.
C'mon.
You're such a dork!
Try again. One more.
Great. You're pulling a knife on me.
Great. You're pulling a knife on me.
Don't even think about repeating everything I say, you dufus.
Okay.

I looked out the window. Thank God. We were already at North Campus, nearly to McIntyre Avenue. The new engineering building, its sun-pierced atrium visible through the high windows in front, blurred past, as did the tall pine trees in front of the physics laboratory. It wouldn't be long before the bus dropped me off at my apartment — or at least to within a short excruciating hop to it. It wouldn't be long before I saw Carrie.

After the waitress left, my mother lectured me about not participating in events we scheduled on John's "off days" — days when he wasn't on the kidney dialysis machine.

"You've known for a week that we were coming here," she said. "You could have picked another day for this clapping business." She said this in front of John, who grimaced and began looking around the room.

My argument was that just being there at Pizza Hut, while I was in the crucial early hours of breaking a world record, was sufficient participation and that sipping a little root beer, under the circumstances, put me solidly in the off-day spirit of things.

She didn't see it that way.

I asked John what he thought. He shook his head; he wanted nothing to do with this conversation.

I kept clapping under the table. Later, after the waitress asked, giggling, if everything was all right with our pizza, I let my mother feed me a bite or two.

HOMAGE TO OLIVER SACKS

*At the very first sign of joint swelling, ACT
IMMEDIATELY! Don't think it is of little
consequence and will soon pass! Don't try to
"get by with it" this time. A joint hemorrhage is a
SERIOUS matter and unless treated immediately
and properly can lead to permanent disability*

— DOROTHY WHITE, *Home Care of the Hemophiliac Child*

A blast of Michigan winter wind startled me as I swung
gingerly down from the bus, Landor's *Imaginary Conversations* tucked under my arm, a corner of Bill Stafford's
letter sticking out of the book's pages like a dorsal fin out of
the ocean. The sun was rising, shimmering off the thin
patches of snow and ice across the parking lot. I hadn't realized how cryptlike the bus felt until I got off. Once I was outside, I was braced by the the cold, sharp-smelling air.

I stared at the grid of cement walks that crisscrossed the
apartment complex. At once I understood vividly the risk I'd
taken by getting back on the bus. Each cement walk was potentially perilous with ice. I should have found another way
to the apartment or, better, gone straight to the emergency
room. But how? Time was of the essence. It's important to get
ice on a bleed as soon as possible. (For the first time I saw the
irony of my needing to treat the bleed with the very substance
that caused it.) Moreover, the sooner you receive an infusion
of factor VIII or DDAVP, the less likely you are to have crippling complications.

I had a history of trying not to involve others in my bleeds, trying not to bother anyone, including Carrie. But of course I needed to bother people, especially Carrie. Years ago I resolved to be more aggressive in treating my bleeds. Looking at the cement walk that led to my apartment, I wondered: *Am I resorting to old habits? Will I go through the familiar process — denial followed by a recognition of my vulnerability and an urgent acceptance that I need help — with each new bleed? Had I started that old process by getting on the bus?*

The apartment wasn't far away — maybe fifty yards. I started toward it, hopping, limping, waddling. I stifled an impulse to yell with pain. Stopping for a moment, standing still in the parking lot, I let the argument with myself play out, trying desperately to determine whether I had done the right thing by getting on the bus. Was I denying my predicament, shirking responsibility for my condition? Had I been reckless or, conversely, recklessly shy?

Each person at the bus stop was utterly preoccupied. Unwilling to have a fissure enter his or her carapace of remoteness and busyness. That was plain as day. Besides, what could they do? Like me, they were waiting for a bus. They weren't in cars. If someone had offered, I'd have accepted a ride.

What about the doctor — or whoever that guy was? You should have asked him for a ride to the emergency room.

I don't know. There was something about him. Would you have trusted your life to that guy?

Well, you should have called Carrie. That's what you should have done. You shouldn't have gotten on that godforsaken bus. Now you have to hop, possibly across ice, possibly causing further damage.

If I'd called Carrie and she wasn't home, then I'd have been stuck. Then I'd have regretted not getting on the bus. You know I'm right about that.

Maybe. Then again, perhaps you're just rationalizing the fact that you screwed up.

I did what I did. Nothing can change it now. Let's just concentrate on getting an infusion and taking care of this.

———

Looking across the parking lot, I could see the basketball court where, three months earlier, I had broken my leg. Leaping to grab a stray rebound, I landed, without the ball, on a stout, rude foot. My ankle turned beneath me. X rays showed a fractured ankle, surprising me and the doctor on call at the emergency room. "Surprising" because the pain was not great, not nearly as great as the pain I was experiencing now, and because the swelling did not result in the usual grotesque sharp-angled hematoma. Each bleed has its own rhythms and manifestations. During convalescence — that is, during the weeks of codeine and waiting for my body to absorb the blood, followed by weeks of physical therapy — one of the books I read was *A Leg to Stand On,* Oliver Sacks's remarkable account of his own experience with a damaged leg, a "neurological novel or short story . . . rooted in personal experience and neurological fact," as Sacks put it. Alone, climbing a mountain in Norway, Sacks encountered a bull, ran blindly from it, and misstepped, severely injuring his left leg. After working for hours to get himself to safety, heaving his leg in front of him as he scooted down the mountain path, he experienced a vivifying revelation:

There came to my aid now melody, rhythm and music (what Kant calls the "quickening" art). Before crossing the stream, I had muscled along — moving by main force, with my very strong arms. Now, so to speak, I was musicked along. I did not contrive this. It happened to me. I fell into a rhythm, guided by a sort of

*marching or rowing song, sometimes the Volga Boat-
men's Song, sometimes a monotonous chant of my
own, accompanied by these words "Ohne Haste, ohne
Rast! Ohne Haste, ohne Rast!" ("Without haste, without rest"), with a strong heave on every* Haste *and*
Rast. . . . *I found myself perfectly co-ordinated by the
rhythm — or perhaps subordinated would be a better
term: the musical beat was generated within me, and
all my muscles responded obediently — all save those in
my left leg, which seemed silent — or mute? . . .*

*Somehow, with this "music," it felt much less like a
grim anxious struggle.*

Yes, I thought when I first read that passage a couple of
months earlier, strung out in bed: *what I need is melody,
rhythm, and music.*

I remembered with keen gratitude the phrase "*musicked
along.*" It mirrored my experience of convalescence, especially
the long, hard hours of physical therapy, grunting and straining
and stretching and strengthening the muscles until they were
once again capable — miraculous! — first of bearing weight and
eventually of coordinated and graceful movement. Listening to
music, or rather *entering* music, letting it inhabit me, participating in it, was crucial to the success of physical therapy,
though I'd never seen anyone acknowledge it before Sacks did.

"Kinetic melody" was another phrase from Sacks's book
that I recalled with gratitude. It referred to the body's instinctive music, its spontaneous kinesthetic precision of muscle
and motion. "Kinetic melody" described in two words what
racing motorcycles, riding skateboards, playing in a band,
taking a walk, as well as convalescence and the desire to push
oneself through grueling physical therapy sessions, were all

about. My body's kinetic melody had been abruptly diminished only minutes ago, yet already I was desperate to rediscover or rehear its full-throated song.

But that would be a long time coming. I knew that. I was a long way from convalescence. First there were dark nights to tremble and thirst through. With the fall on the ice, I had taken up residence for a while in, to borrow a line of Sylvia Plath's, "a country as far away as health," which at the moment seemed the exact distance to the front door of my apartment. Looking at the fifty yards in front of me, wondering how to traverse it without further injury, it indeed appeared that I was in for a "grim anxious struggle." I felt as though I were trapped in Zeno's dichotomy paradox, wherein travel from one point in space to another is impossible because each step toward the second point involves traveling half the distance to that point, and then half that distance, and half that distance again, and so on, ad infinitum. I hoped to invoke music (though not, please God, the "Song of the Volga Boatmen") in order to "music along" and overcome the seemingly infinite distance.

There came to my aid now the Clash — in particular the Clash's manic, searing, magisterial recording, on the album *London Calling*, of "Brand New Cadillac." In my mind I replayed again and again Mick Jones's opening solo riffs and the major chord, the snarling major chord, the band joins in with. The music is thrillingly alive and resonant. My body translated that resonance into its own odd music as I hopped and limped and waddled, but rhythmically, around icy stretches of cement toward my apartment. The rhythm of the guitars quickened me. The song's fierceness entered me. There was no longer any doubt about my making it to the apartment without falling again. I felt within my body the "certain primitive exuberance" that Sacks felt as he heaved his damaged leg down the mountain trail.

The Clash burst open the desolate trap of Zeno's paradox. Music flooded inside.

———

At last I was at the front door.

I had guessed correctly: Carrie was working at the computer when I shoved open the door and hopped in, grimacing and grabbing my leg. The computer sat on an old oak library table against the far wall of the living room. Carrie heard me enter and turned around to say hello.

She took one look at me and said, "You're having a bleed."

Nov. 27, 1972

Dear Tom,

Today, I was really shocked while listening to an after-noon radio program — here in Las Vegas.

The MC of this program has a quiz every afternoon & gives a free record album to the one who answers the question. Today, his question was —

What did Tom Andrews of Charleston, West Virginia, do for 14 hours & some minutes that is a world record?

Well, Tom, I got so excited because he went on to say that Tom was 11 years old & I just knew it had to be you. I was so flustered that I couldn't think what you might have done — so I decided to call my answer in that you had walked that long in the Polio March. I told the master of ceremonies that I had known an 11-year-old Tom Andrews, that we had gone to the same church, etc. The fellow thought it a coincidence that someone here would know this young man, & he said he would give me an album because I had known you. Of course, I can't accept it until I know that it really was the Tom I knew.

Are you the boy who clapped his hands for over 14 hours?

If not, it doesn't matter, as it has been nice writing to you.

Charlie Bob (we call him CB now) has really enjoyed the desert, as have we all. There are so many interesting things to see that are new to us. He sends you a big hello.

Would you like to know some of the answers that were called in? One man, a Mr. Throckmorton, guessed the handclapping. Some of the others said—

1. *Mountain climbing*
2. *Jumping on pogo stick*
3. *Taking a 14-hour shower*
4. *Shoveling coal*
5. *Bike racing*
6. *Playing Ping-Pong*

Please give my regards to your mother, & we will be anxious to know if we really know the holder of a world record!

Your friend,
Mrs. C. L. Showalter

LET US NOW PRAISE
FAMOUS WOMEN

With each accident, there is a moment when I see Carrie for the first time after the bleeding begins, and each time I know I'll never in my life be happier to see her. But each new bleed makes that prior knowledge obsolete. As this one did.

Carrie! Her precious narrow face, thin nose, hazel-flecked-with-green irises, long henna-blond hair. When I left her in the morning to catch the bus, she was wearing a white flannel nightgown wrinkled from sleep. Now she was wearing baggy blue jeans and a rust-colored wool sweater.

I sat down on the floor, propping my leg up with pillows gathered from surrounding chairs so that my ankle was higher than my head. I set *Imaginary Conversations* on the floor beside me, relieved that it and Stafford's letter had survived the morning's journey intact. Immediately Carrie put some ice in a plastic sandwich bag, wrapped the bag in a washcloth, and handed it to me. I wanted to take my shoe off but remembered the good advice the ersatz doctor had given me about my ankle's swelling "like a mother." I decided to wait until I got to the emergency room. I rolled down my sock and looked at the swelling. Yes, there was a tennis-ball-sized knot of flesh sitting on top of the anklebone, poking out grotesquely, seeming to strain the elasticity of the skin. The skin was deep red, and it was hot. It was burning up. I placed — *careful* — the ice on the swollen, seething knot.

Carrie got ready to take me to the emergency room. I began describing, as best I could, what had happened. It was difficult to speak coherently. I described falling on the ice, lying there with my back on the sidewalk by the Rackham Building, seeing for an instant the glistening bare trees and the yew bushes and beyond them a clear blue winter sky. I described the Clash's role in getting me from the parking lot to the front door. I described the conversations on the bus. I described my thoughts about John and imitated John's deadpan voice: "Great. You're pulling a knife on me."

"You should write this stuff down," Carrie said as she rushed through the apartment finding things I would need at the hospital.

"And," I said, closing my eyes quickly, as if that would help diminish the throbbing in my leg, "I just met Doogie Howser's big brother."

"Who?" Carrie called out from the bedroom.

"You know, that precocious kid who's a doctor in a TV series. *Doogie Howser, M.D.* The kid I met was big, though. He had lug nuts in his neck. Never mind. I'm just talking. Thanks for, you know, doing this."

Carrie appeared from the bedroom with her keys in one hand and an overstuffed paper bag in the other. The bag jutted out at sharp angles and points; I knew it was full of books. "Ready?" Carrie asked. "Wait. I'll get your crutches."

———

Carrie helped me to the car, a gas-guzzling Buick built during the Kennedy administration, and into the backseat, where I could stretch out my leg. I was headed to the emergency room at last. I looked at my watch: a quarter after nine. It had been about thirty-five minutes since the accident. The timing was not ideal, but it was all right, on the whole.

After hearing my story, Carrie was upset. "Why didn't you call me? Honestly. Hopping like that. *Hopping*." She glanced at me through the rearview mirror.

I sank wearily into the car seat. I replayed for her the argument I had had with myself. "I decided that if you weren't here, I'd have been in worse trouble."

Carrie was upset, but she was also a model of intelligent concern. Over the years she had developed a no-nonsense approach to bleeds, an approach that calmed me and, paradoxically, gave me the freedom to occasionally "catastrophize," as psychological counselors put it, uttering worst-case scenarios out loud to get them out of my head. I didn't indulge in such utterances now. Carrie was articulating her dismay.

"Sometimes I think you *want* to have complications. To punish yourself."

"Punish myself? For what?" I strained to hear each syllable, each scrap of meaning in her voice.

"For — I don't know. Maybe I shouldn't say this. Not now. I'm sorry."

"No, what? It's okay. Go ahead." I meant it. I welcomed this sudden plunge into uncomfortable honesty. It mimicked my leg's plunge into another kind of uncomfortable honesty. Apparently Carrie had been hoarding something inside her for a while; I was pleased to give her a chance to clear the air.

"I just think, sometimes, you've never forgiven yourself for surviving. While, you know, John didn't."

Relief came over me. Carrie was right, but she wasn't saying anything I hadn't thought of myself.

"I think you're right," I said. "I mean, I know you're right." I shook my head. "Boy, am I relieved. I was sure you thought I wanted to punish myself for having had impure thoughts about Ruth Buzzi."

Dead silence. The silence of unlaughter.

Carrie gave me a look of pure incomprehension and pity. It was the kind of look that made me think it was a miracle on par with the discovery of Neptune's rings that Carrie had ever agreed to marry me.

"Sorry," I mumbled into my leg. I adjusted the ice bag. My leg seethed.

"That's okay," Carrie said. "I knew this wasn't the time to get into anything." She stared fixedly at the road. For the third time in the space of an hour, I passed the various academic buildings of North Campus, their lawns of slush and brown grass. We headed for Fuller Avenue and Medical Center Drive.

"It wasn't a *bad* joke," Carrie said at last, extinguishing the long silence, grinning. "But, just a tip, wincing doesn't do much for your delivery."

I looked at Carrie and smiled. This last comment was a gift. I took it gratefully, wordlessly. I took a rest from words, tried to empty my mind of them, until we got to the emergency room.

The emergency room at the University of Michigan Hospital is like the entrance to a Hyatt Regency. You half expect valet parking. Mercifully easy of access, unconfusing, it was designed for persons in urgent need. I confess to years of evil wishes for the architects of hospitals as I was taxied in circles looking for the emergency-room entrance. The poet Louis Zukofsky wrote that modern architecture exists in order "to make it more ugly to the airport." The University of Michigan Hospital contradicts that statement absolutely. It sets a corrective, blessedly anomalous standard.

Carrie helped me out of the car. A vigorous-looking elderly man in a blue hospital volunteer jacket stood beside an empty wheelchair; he had just wheeled another patient to a waiting car. He offered the wheelchair to us and adjusted the right leg assembly so that my leg would be elevated. "There you go," he said jovially, patting the wheelchair. "This one belongs in a museum, but it'll get you where you want to go." Carrie pushed me through the door, past the waiting area, and toward the admissions desk.

At once I smelled the familiar, funereal, ammonia-laden odor of hospitals.

———————

Carrie wheeled me to the admissions desk. There I was met by a smiling, pleasant-voiced woman in a pink frilly dress. She wore braces that covered both of her wrists and forearms. The name of her condition escaped me; then it was on the tip of my tongue; then I had it. Tarpal cunnel syndrome. No. Carpal tunnel syndrome.

"Carpal tunnel?" I asked.

"The doctor thinks so," she said. "These things sure help. That's for sure." She lifted her hands from her computer keyboard and wiggled her fingers, as if to say, "See?"

"Good," I said.

Carrie, who had been standing behind me, whispered, "I'm going to go park the car, Tom. I'll be right back."

"Okay," I said. "I'll be here."

By the time Carrie traced her steps back to the waiting area, I realized I'd forgotten to call *MR* and the English department. "Carrie!" I yelled. Carrie turned around in a panic. I said, "I forgot to call work. I'm supposed to teach today. Would you call *MR,* it doesn't matter who you talk to, and Janet, the secretary of the English department? Janet will put a note on the door of my classroom."

Carrie sighed visibly. "Yes, okay, but don't scare me like that! They'll have to put *me* in here." Then she was through the waiting area and out the door.

The woman at the admissions desk asked me for my insurance card. I gave it gladly. Though I made almost nothing, only

$12,500, at *Mathematical Reviews,* I had excellent medical coverage through the University of Michigan's insurance system. It was comprehensive, even to employees like me with expensive preexisting conditions, and remarkably hassle-free. The insurance horror stories many hemophiliacs lived out were enough to make me determined to stay at *MR* for as long as I could stand editing mathematical texts that, as Walter liked to joke, were too complicated for God *or* the Devil to figure out.

While the pleasant-voiced woman at the admissions desk punched some numbers into her computer, I removed my right shoe and sock. I felt a dizzying rush of blood into the hollow just under the anklebone; the hollow seemed to fill up like an ink sponge. I opened my mouth, Munch-like, to cry out but kept quiet. The woman looked up from her computer, saw the grotesque knot growing out of my ankle, and gasped.

That *she* would react that way — she who no doubt witnessed each day an unthinkable parade of misery and malady — was curiously, or perversely, reassuring. It meant I wasn't crazy to be so alarmed and disoriented. Genuine human responses, such as an involuntary gasp, are in short supply among hospital staff. This woman's candor brought a split second of relief.

The woman regained her professional demeanor and said, "I bet that hurts."

"Yes," I said, nodding.

"What should I put down as the problem?" she asked.

I distilled the story to its emergency-room essence: *I'm a hemophiliac, I fell on ice, I'm having a bleed, I need an infusion of DDAVP.*

"Hemo . . . philiac," she said, typing the word. "And you've been to this emergency room before?"

"Oh, yes," I said. "Three months ago, in fact."

"My, my," she said. "You just can't stay away from our hospitality, can you?"

I smiled grimly.

She took the grimness of my smile as a signal that I was no longer up to exchanging pleasantries. She stiffened professionally.

"Any allergies?"

"No."

She raised her eyebrows, continuing to type. "You're not allergic to penicillin?"

"No."

She seemed pleased for me, proud that my system tolerated penicillin. "Good!" she said. Under different circumstances, I would have asked why she reacted this way. Was she being sarcastic? But now, I thought, *Whatever.*

"Are you presently taking any medication?"

"No."

She asked me to hold out my left wrist, on which she affixed the hospital identification bracelet. "Now don't take that off," she said. "You can wait right over there till you're called." She pointed to the waiting area.

I wheeled myself over there. It was nearly empty. One other family, or what I assumed to be a family—a woman and man and a boy with Down's syndrome—was waiting to be called. The man was bald and sweaty, and hefty, and I think he was drunk. The woman swam inside her large leather coat. She suffered the man, who seemed to be pleading with her. The boy was sitting in a chair across from me. His knees were drawn up to his chest. He rocked back and forth, muttering, "I want to go. I want to go. I want to go." He turned his broad, short head from side to side. The man and woman, immersed in their dispiriting exchange, were oblivious to the boy. The boy looked at me and said, "I want to go. I want to go."

"I want to go, too," I said.

In front of me, beyond the boy and the waiting area, were several plywood partitions blocking off a part of the hospital that was being renovated. I could see through a gap in the partitions. The ceiling was very high, and the cement walls were unpainted. Tools lay here and there. At the moment no one was working on it. It was dimly lit. It looked like one of the bleak industrial sets in Terry Gilliam's movie *Brazil,* the visual imagery of which had fascinated me, though I didn't want to let it become a metaphor for my time in the hospital.

A nurse walked into the waiting area and called aloud the boy's name. "Come on, honey," said the woman beside the boy, taking him by the hand as she stood up. The man stood up, too, and all of them vanished behind the admissions desk, into the examination area.

———

I needed an infusion. I wanted to withdraw into myself like the boy, rock back and forth and mutter, "I need an infusion. I need an infusion. I need an infusion." For what seemed a long time I didn't see another soul. My leg—now the calf as well as the ankle—drilled into itself like an auger. My head dangled loosely onto my chest. The objects nearest me — tables, chairs, walls, a Coke machine, tiles embedded in the floor—threatened to erase themselves, threadbare sketches drawn in invisible ink. I was entering a suction of hysteria and dread. I closed my eyes, hoping to stave off sinking further into this abysmal moment. Worse times were ahead, I knew. If I lost my edge of clarity at this early stage, I hadn't a prayer of keeping my sanity through the weeks ahead.

Focus. I uttered aloud a line from a Bill Stafford poem: "Treat the world as if it really existed." *Yes. Incline heart and mind to the real. Incline, Tom, incline!*

I remembered the "reality orientation" exercises I'd occasionally led patients through at Holland Community Hospital, where I worked as a volunteer in the psychiatric ward and emergency room the summer I graduated from Hope College. *Your name is — ? The date is — ? The weather is — ? Tomorrow is — ? Your birthday is — ? You were born in the city of — ?* I felt silly even thinking to ask myself these questions. The feeling of silliness, in turn, convinced me that I was not on the verge of hysteria after all. Nevertheless, my eyes remained closed.

I tried to invoke music again, fill my inner ear with "Brand New Cadillac" or the Gang of Four's "Not Great Men" (another favorite) or any estranged snatch of song. This time nothing answered the call. I was learning again that I could not *decide* to hear music while my leg pulsed with the eloquence of a hammer blow to the nerve endings. Whatever music — or image, or voice — arrived, arrived involuntarily, beyond will or misgiving, startling in its abruptness. Again I heard John's tremulous voice, rehearsing from his sweet oblivion a running argument we'd had years ago:

Elvis Costello is fifty, no, a hundred times more talented than Elvis Presley. There's no comparison.

Get a life, Tom. I can't believe what I'm hearing.

Seriously. Talent-wise, Elvis Costello owns the rights to the name Elvis.

You're such an idiot! He wouldn't even have the name Elvis *if it weren't for Elvis Presley. This is such a stupid conversation. You know that Elvis Costello isn't his real name. You know that, don't you?*

Yeah, yeah. Big deal. Declan McManus. His real name's Declan McManus.

59

Tell me, why do you think he chose the name Elvis?

Because of Elvis Presley. Of course. Granted. That's not the argument. The argument is that he eclipsed his namesake.

This is hopeless. Tell me you're joking.

Here. Put on any Elvis Presley record. Then let me play "Watching the Detectives" or "Radio, Radio" or "Pump It Up." I'll make a believer out of you.

You've made a believer out of me. I believe that you have tin ears and nothing between them.

The Great Elvis Debate brought to mind—mercifully—another long-running shtick John and I often fell into when he was on dialysis or when either of us was in the hospital. We called it "Laurel and Hardy: An Oral Hystery." John played Oliver Hardy. I was Stan Laurel. John was too uncoordinated to physically reenact scenes from the films, so we pretended to be Laurel and Hardy in retirement, undergoing an interminable nostalgic interview with a Leonard Maltin–like journalist/admirer. We memorized actual interviews, gathered from biographies such as John McCabe's *Mr. Laurel and Mr. Hardy,* and took turns playing the interviewer. We loved sneaking into the auditorium at Morris Harvey College (now the University of Charleston); looking out over row after row of crushed red velvet seats, we pretended the interview took place in front of a standing-room-only crowd.

> INTERVIEWER: Babe, tell us how you came to twiddle your tie. When was the first time?
>
> HARDY: Yes, well, it was in a silent called *Why Girls Love Sailors.* I got splashed in the face with a bucket —
>
> LAUREL: Actually, it was in *Sailors Beware.*
>
> HARDY: Do you mind? I got splashed in the face with a bucket of water. I'm sure this was in *Why Girls*

Love Sailors. I was expecting the splash, and yet in a way I wasn't. It threw me mentally, just for a second or so, and I just couldn't think of what to do next. The camera was grinding away and I knew I had to do *something,* so I thought of blowing my nose with my wet and sopping tie. I was raising my tie to my nose when I realized that this would be a bit vulgar. There were some ladies watching us. So I waved the tie in a kind of tiddly-widdly fashion, in a kind of comic way, to show that I was embarrassed.

The memory of these deadpan sessions brought a few precious seconds of distraction. I kept my eyes shut, fearful that everything in my visual field would become ghostly and insubstantial, a loose skein unwinding madly, if I opened them. The memory of "Laurel and Hardy: An Oral Hystery" quickly turned sour. How different were those blithe performances from the conversations John and I had had during his last fundamentalist-evangelical years. During that time, John would "witness" to me ("In witnessing," he wrote in a notebook, "silence isn't always GOLDEN, sometimes it's just plain YELLOW!") and mourn that I wouldn't be with him on the Shores of Glory.

Somewhere within that tortured and fearful rhetoric was a viable faith for John. I wanted to understand it. I wanted to investigate it with sympathy. But thinking about it nearly overwhelmed me with grief.

————

Think of something else.
Where was Carrie?

————

I decided that Carrie was probably on the phone, talking to Janet at the English department or Nancy or Terry at *MR*. My spirits lifted a bit at the thought of Terry and her response to news of my accident. She didn't treat my bleeds as if they represented the end of the world. She was sympathetic, helpful, and altogether ruthless with jokes. Three months earlier, when I broke my ankle playing basketball, she had placed a new nameplate on my desk:

TOM ANDREWS, CRAZED BLEEDER JOCK

To Terry, a hemophiliac playing basketball was exhibiting suicidal tendencies. "Then I don't have to ask what you think about a hemo racing motorcycles," I said to her. "No points for guessing that one," she said. This time I could look Terry in the eye and say that the only high-risk activity I was indulging in was riding the bus.

Blood ballooned miserably into my leg. My leg throbbed with each pulse. I actually thought I could see my pulse, pounding stubbornly, when I looked at the swollen calf and ankle.

It helped to think of my colleagues at *MR*. They made up a remarkable collection of oddballs and visionaries. I felt enormous affection for them, perhaps because for the first time in my life I worked with people more eccentric than myself. Nearly all the senior editors were extraplanetary, bespectacled men and women so caught up in the inward bank and shoal of mathematical experience that they bumped into one another in the hallways, each truly amazed that the building had other inhabitants. The copyeditors watched this "Keystone Kops Meet Pythagoras" routine play out on a daily basis, and felt superior. We may not be likely to prove Fermat's Last Theorem (the elusive proof that there do not exist whole numbers X, Y, and Z such that $X^N + Y^N = Z^N$ for some number N greater than 2), we thought, but at least we knew how to get in and out of the grocery store. One editor told me he had figured out a route to and from work each day that involved making only right-angled turns. The copyeditors howled when I reported that one. I would sorely miss them during the two months it would take my leg to absorb the blood and regain strength enough to allow me to return to the office.

Still in the waiting area, I imagined the daily fugue of voices in the Wormhole, voices lofted into that shared humming space while the Fuzzy Sets poured over mathematical obscurities:

> "*Listen to these adjectives*. A charged particle damped anharmonic nonlinear oscillator motion. *Six, count 'em, six adjectives!*"

> "*That's nothing, listen to this.* A finite state finite action infinite discrete time horizon Markov decision process. *That's, let's see, nine . . . ten adjectives.* Ten. *That's a record. Isn't that a record?*"

> "*What day does the first day of spring fall on this year? A Monday?*"

> "*I got a new sci-fi novel today. It's about post-nuke Mormonism.*"

> "*Here's a title for you, Mark. 'Escape and Capture in the Restricted Three-Body Problem.'*"

> "*My three-body problems are all unrestricted, ha-ha-ha.*"

> "*Why is it everything you say has white American male stamped all over it in boldface?*"

> "*Eighteen-point italic, you mean.*"

"Did you know that in Chinese it's easy to say, 'You are a turtle's egg,' when you mean, 'How are you'?"

Freewheeling talk was a compensation we allotted one another for being strangers in the strange land of professional mathematics. Another was our palpable amazement at the minds whose brilliant scratches and indecipherable markings we edited. At least, that was the case with me. Though I was not a gifted mathematician, I learned to recognize a beautiful theorem when one crossed my desk, and I was awestruck. Awe disclosed to me what I could not otherwise understand.

I tried to recall a theorem, but it was hopeless. Blood pressed against the nerve endings in my ankle and calf. Pain ground its teeth. I needed help quickly. There was no way around it. My leg was damaged. I was bleeding. I couldn't distract my mind any longer. The bleeding had to be stopped.

The bleeding had to be stopped.

In 1972 I was a fifth grader at Oakwood Elementary School in the South Hills section of Charleston. November 15 was a Wednesday, but it was a day devoted to conferences between parents and teachers, and the students had the day off. My mother had scheduled conferences with John's teachers in the morning and with mine in the late afternoon. Before she left to meet John's teachers, perhaps just around the time when her initial dismay at my clapping began changing to resignation that she had in fact raised a complete idiot, she walked into the "green room" — the room where we kept John's dialysis machine and the television and my father's stereo system. John and I sat on the sofa watching The Price Is Right. *We had the volume turned up so we could hear Bob Barker above the sound of my clapping. My mother had been in the kitchen, thinking about the spiritual delinquencies of her children.*

She looked at John and me staring at the TV. I looked up at her. She had curly brown hair and wide glasses with brown frames.

"Tell me this, Tom," she said. Her voice was grave and direct. "Are you doing this for God's glory or your own?"

"God's," I said automatically.

Bob Barker smooched the wife of a man who had just won a camper and a Yamaha dirt bike.

"Uh-huh," my mother said.

I lied, of course.

I tried to shrug off my mother's question. But it got to me. I was deeply ashamed of the worldly ambition my record represented. When the record appeared a year later, several classmates at Oakwood came up to me holding hardcover copies of The Guinness Book of World Records *and asked if that was really me who had clapped my hands.*

"Oh, no," I explained. "My brother's the one who broke the record. But there was a horrible mix-up, and they printed my name *instead. Boy, is he pissed!"*

SLOUCHING TOWARDS CODEINE

*Any university doctor is an armed and shielded
giant, against whom the defenseless body-dwarf
cannot do battle.*

— GUIDO CERONETTI

An incendiary jolt through my leg. The heat cranked up
a notch. I twisted in the wheelchair. All it took was
one such jolt, and my equilibrium collapsed entirely. Suddenly I was again beset by questions, some reasonable, some
irrational and childish. They whirled through my head like
tiny snowflakes in a vigorously shaken glass globe. I closed
my eyes.

*Will the emergency-room doctor be familiar with DDAVP?
Has it been too long since the accident to avoid permanent
damage to the joint's cartilage? Will the leg ever heal? Will I
be able to run again? Walk without a limp?*

*Will my insurance cover everything? What if my insurance
company decides I am too expensive and stops paying? Or
starts charging outrageously high premiums, as has happened
with other hemophiliacs I know? Why have I been so lucky so
far — with insurance, with my cartilage, with HIV? Is my
number up, has my luck run out?*

*Since I've had so many bleeds in this ankle, will the joint
have to be fused?* (The procedure is called arthrodesis, by
which a chronically damaged joint is immobilized by fusing
the bones together and removing painful joint tissues. After
my previous bleed, my hematologist had discussed with me

the possibility of fusing my right ankle.) *Will I have to argue with my hematologist against fusion?*

––––––––

The sound of an elevator door opening behind me. I heard blind, hurried footsteps: frenzy declared by the feet. I opened my eyes. The image of a grief-stricken man in a gray suit charging toward the admissions desk did not threaten to disappear, did not erase itself. I saw this man. Big athletic build, wide back, blank ashen face. I saw him. Something, some elusive motion of spirit (fellow feeling I think to call it now), was made clear to me, and I was humbled by it. *How unwavering and purposeful is the man's body,* I thought. *How bravely and tenaciously it carries the wreckage of fear, need, circumstance.*

Of course, I knew nothing about his fear or need or circumstance. My fellow feeling did not console or ease his obvious burden, practically or in any other way, in the least. All the same, my heart expanded and broke for this man, for his brave, burdened steps echoing throughout the waiting room. His raw grief, his frenzied footsteps were part of the huge world beyond my puny self.

––––––––

The nurse I'd seen earlier walked up to my wheelchair and said, "Mr. Andrews?"

"Yes," I said. "That's me."

The nurse wheeled me past the admissions desk to a table in the examination area. Drawing the privacy curtain, she said, "Let's get you up on the scales."

This was a good sign. Weighing me meant she was thinking about allotting the right amount of clotting factor for my body weight. It made me think she had dealt with hemophiliacs before.

She removed the bag of ice from my ankle, set it on the counter by the sink, and gripped me under my arms. With her support, I rose from the wheelchair, trying not to show on my face the predictable delirium of pain shooting through my leg. The nurse maneuvered me onto the scales and weighed me. I felt like a brook trout in a fishnet. Did I weigh enough, or would she be required to throw me back into the Huron River?

"One thirty-eight," she said to her clipboard. "Nothing but skin and bones."

She was about to help me into the wheelchair when she paused. I watched her ask herself a question. Which would be less painful: easing him back into the wheelchair and wheeling him the ten feet to the examination table, or having him hop the ten feet on his good leg?

"Never mind the wheelchair," I said. "I'm already up."

The nurse helped me onto the table and replaced the ice bag. She took my temperature and blood pressure, both of which were fine. "The doctor will be right with you," she said, ducking behind the privacy curtain.

I was alone again for a little while.

During recent bleeds, as pain descended upon and inhabited me, I worked hard to remind myself that my body was more than simply the damaged limb or bloated nerve-tossed joint. I needed to remind myself of this now. I was not all leg. My leg was "me" — that is, its daily function and coordination played a surprisingly large role in my understanding of myself — but I was not *all* leg. But how to convince myself of that when pain insisted otherwise?

Pain brought me — as it would several times before I left the hospital — to the threshold of a kind of ontological breakdown. As blood drained away into the flushed interior of my leg, I grew strange to myself, alienated from whatever self I used to answer to. Before the bleed, I moved and lived within a relation to myself, as described wonderfully by Gerard Manley Hopkins:

> *my self-being, my consciousness and feeling of myself, that taste of myself, of I and me . . . which is more distinctive than the taste of ale or alum, more distinctive than the smell of walnutleaf or camphor . . .*

During the bleed, nothing was less distinctive than the taste of myself. The taste was like that of a stale communion wafer, one that offered no hope of transubstantiation.

Again I uttered aloud the line of Bill Stafford's. "Treat the world as if it really existed." *Concentrate on other stimuli,* I said to myself. *What, besides the pain in your leg, are you experiencing right now, right this second?*

Always there was the hospital's pungent smell, the smell of unguents and antiseptics, perfuming illness as though it were a fetid body.

I looked around the examination area. Every inch of available space was being used to store medical equipment and appliances. I made an inventory. There was a shining Hewlett-Packard defibrillator (Code Master XL +), whatever that was. There were Silvon diaphoretic ECG electrodes. There were suture trays and boxes of vinyl examination gloves (Correct Touch, X-Large). There was an X-ray reading panel. There was a suction catheter with DeLee tip (manufactured by the Argyle Company). There was a Shadowless Skytron light (Vamada Shadowless Lamp Co.). There were boxes of Pre-Op II iodophor surgical scrub sponges and bags of Baxter 1000 ml 0.9% sodium chloride injection USP. There were oxygen masks with eighty-four-inch tubing. There was an AMSC warming cabinet. There was a laundry hamper. There were—

An unsteady hand drew open the privacy curtain, inter-rupting my inventory.

Carrie!

"I wasn't sure which curtain was yours," Carrie said. "I ac-cidentally peeked in on a woman changing her clothes." She was carrying her leather purse and the bag of books I'd seen her carry out of the apartment.

"Have you seen the doctor yet?" she asked.

In the fifteen or so minutes since I'd last seen Carrie, it felt as if a whole phase of the moon had passed. There was no way to tell her about all the hesitations and impressions and memories I'd experienced in such a short time: the di-versionary tactics my mind came up with, the memories of affections, the half-perceived revelations, the dread, the bucking up. Each second had seemed fraught with crucial significance. Had her experience been similar? I was frus-trated that the best I could do was construct a kind of scrim through which she could faintly glimpse the fullness of what I was not able to describe. I was frustrated, too, that I would be able to glimpse the richness of *her* experience only through a similar scrim. The mismatched wedding of language and consciousness never felt more capricious or sadistic.

I told Carrie all this, and she said, "Write it down. Just write it down. Have you seen the doctor yet?"

"No," I said. "I saw the nurse not long before you got here. She said the doctor would be here in a minute."

"Right. In a minute," Carrie said sarcastically just as the curtain rattled open and a young doctor appeared, his pink, lean face runneled and pocked with acne. "Dr. Andrews?" he asked. The respect in his voice surprised me.

I smiled appreciatively. "I'm afraid only one of those two words is correct," I said.

The young doctor looked confused. Immediately I worried that we were getting off to a bad start. *It can't be a good sign,* I thought, *to confuse your doctor before he even looks at you.*

The first meeting with a doctor always feels to me like the first awkward moments of a blind date. You're nervous, you're trying to appear calm, and you're hoping to score points with humor or thoughtfulness or exaggerated listening skills. As soon as the doctor opened the curtain to my space in the emergency room, I seemed to be losing points on all counts.

Maybe I should have pretended to have a Ph.D.? I tried conversational backpedaling. "I mean, thank you for being generous," I offered sheepishly.

"I see," the young doctor said, looking at my chart. "Since you work at *Mathematical Reviews* and teach at the U, I assumed you had your Ph.D."

The balloon of his respect for me deflated.

"No," I said, "but I've been reading without moving my lips since I turned twenty-seven."

Where did I think I was, a lodge in the Catskills? I was in no shape to tell jokes. My body pleaded with me to speak as little as possible, and yet I couldn't stop until I received a signal that I was entertaining this dour young acne-ridden doctor, wooing him, making him like me, gaining back the ground I had lost for being a putz with an M.F.A. I tried again.

"I can juggle. Does that count?"

What was I doing? Carrie looked embarrassed for me. She reached for my hand and held it consolingly.

"Count?" the young doctor asked distractedly, avoiding eye contact. His eyebrows came together.

I felt ashamed for sucking up to him. Then I felt anger for feeling ashamed. Why did these emotional booby traps appear during bleeds? It occurred to me that a healthier response would have been to rip the stethoscope from the doctor's neck, stretch it back like a rubber band, and—*Hello, planet Earth calling! It was just a dumb passive-aggressive joke!*—snap the chart out of his hands, the way sharpshooters in Hollywood westerns shot the gun out of a rival's grip.

This is utterly ridiculous, I told myself. You shouldn't care what the doctor thinks of you. You always go through this. You're not here to entertain him. It's his job to relieve your suffering. If he acts like a jerk, big deal, so you won't invite him over for a beer.

I calmed down, but the pain did not relent. Blood pumped relentlessly, a slow-moving piston, against the insides of my knee, calf, and ankle. I realized that I was trying to make the doctor fall in love with me to ensure that he would give me codeine.

Of all the transactions I've had over the years with doctors, the ugliest and most humiliating by far have been those concerning pain and pain medication. There is a ruthless dialectic at work in the transaction. The hemophiliac with a bleeding joint wants immediate relief; by the time he arrives at the hospital, the pain is often literally unspeakable, beyond utterance. Its wordlessness, however, is precisely what can make the doctor conservative with medication. Emergency-room doctors are used to patients howling with pain, even being deranged by it. If a patient is not howling or screaming, but at the same time not able to speak coherently about what he or she is suffering (sometimes one can speak coherently about anything *but* the pain), it's easy for the doctor to assume pain is not a priority.

"[T]he pain of a bleeding joint is one of the worst known to medical science," Suzanne Massie wrote in *Journey*. But a bleeding joint may not look especially painful. The doctor must rely on the patient to articulate the pain—at the very moment when the patient often retreats far from language. If the patient does not howl and scream, how is the doctor to understand? The patient cannot articulate the pain; the doctor cannot see it. Then again, if the patient *is* able to find language, however inadequate, for his or her suffering, the doctor may take that very articulateness as a sign that the pain must not be as bad as the patient is letting on. Add to all this the fact that doctors (being well aware that hemophiliacs can become addicted to their painkillers) need to be cautious when prescribing addictive drugs such as codeine, Darvon, Demerol, and Percodan, and you see the dilemma.

At such times I do my best to convince the doctor that the pain is awful — usually by grunts and groans. It is a humiliating negotiation. Sometimes the doctor understands right away and prescribes serious pain medication. Other times the doctor is skeptical and prescribes acetaminophen, which is useless. You feel the doctor's intense gaze, doubting you, wondering why your pain threshold is so low. You try again to make the doctor understand: more grunts. The doctor says, *Yes, yes, I understand,* but the prescription stays the same. You argue, using whatever methods are available to you. You become a "difficult" patient. The doctor winces. The prescription stays the same. You become enraged at the dynamic of power you're caught in. The doctor thinks — you can see the thoughts rising like cartoon balloons — the doctor thinks, *It doesn't look so bad, I have certain criteria to consider, I have certain standards, no one tells me what pain medication to administer, don't be a troublemaker, don't be a wussy, I'm the voice of reason around here.* The prescription stays the same.

The transaction ends — quickly or after some time, depending on the emergency-room doctor — with Carrie or a nurse calling Sheryl, the hemophilia nurse coordinator at the University of Michigan Hospital. Sheryl quickly finds a hematologist, and he or she phones in a prescription for codeine. (For some reason codeine, though not as strong as some of the other analgesics, works best for me. Darvon makes me nauseous and dizzy; Demerol makes me nauseous and sweaty; Percodan gives me the "spins" and headaches. Morphine works best, but I find it powerfully addictive; I try not to use it except in the absolute worst case.)

What kind of scene would play itself out with this young doctor, God help him? I wanted codeine now, and I wanted to avoid conflict in getting it. I had not retreated far from language; I had retreated into an absurd language of bad jokes, thinking to woo him. As I watched him inspect my ankle and calf and knee, my spirits plummeted at the thought that I had made a terrible error. Now, I assumed, I would never get an adequate painkiller.

"How's it feel?" the doctor asked, his right forefinger pressing very gently against the swollen knot on my ankle. The knot was now plum-colored. It went white when he pressed on it, then quickly returned to plum when he removed his finger. It was still very hot. "Not too bad, I hope."

"It's not good," I said. I tried to make my voice sound as dispassionate as possible. "It's really bad."

"Really?" he asked.

I thought I heard derision in his repetition of *really*.

"Yes, really," I said.

(Had I said it too sharply? Did it sound as whiny to him as it did to me? Had I offended him? What's the matter with me? I've given up bad jokes for the language of paranoia—always an attractive conversational ploy.)

Carrie saw a standoff approaching and stepped in to intercept it. "Show him the letters," she said.

"Oh yeah," I said. I extracted two well-creased letters from my wallet and handed them to the young doctor. I carry the letters in my wallet for just such an occasion. The first letter, written by Sheryl, is addressed to emergency-room doctors. Sheryl wrote the letter so I could educate the doctors — tactfully, without appearing to — on the proper dosage and preparation of DDAVP, which most of them are unfamiliar with. "This way," Sheryl said when she gave me the letter during one of my checkups, "the doctor doesn't have to suffer the indignity of being taught by a patient." Sheryl's brand of *realpolitik* comforted me. "And," she added, "all *you* have to do is produce the letter — at a time when you probably don't feel like explaining anything to anybody."

The doctor took the first letter and read it.

Should Mr. Andrews experience bleeding of a non-life-threatening nature which requires treatment, the treatment product of choice is desmopressin acetate (DDAVP, Stimate) at a dose of 0.3 micrograms per kilogram given intravenously in 50 ml of normal saline over 20–30 minutes. Desmopressin acetate stimulates the release of factor VIII from endothelial storage sites and causes a transient rise of circulating factor VIII. . . . If follow-up doses are required, this dosage can be repeated in 8 hours. Further repeating of doses is not indicated, as storage sites become depleted.

Life-threatening bleeding should not be treated with desmopressin acetate, but with the purest factor concentrate available.

The second letter narrated for the doctor the terse autobiography of my blood:

Factor VIII assay	<3%
Factor VIII inhibitor	none present
White blood cells	7400
Red blood cells	5.30
Hemoglobin	16.6
Hematocrit	47.1
Platelets	296,000
SGOT	30
SGPT	22
LDH	178

"This is really interesting," the doctor said after reading the letters. I made a mental note to thank Sheryl the next time I saw her. "We'll set up an IV with the DDAVP, but it may take a little while for the pharmacy to make it. In the meantime, we'll need some X rays of your ankle. It looks like there may be a fracture. I recommend staying here in the hospital until the bleeding stops. I've called upstairs—there's a room waiting for you. And I'll get you something for the pain right away. What's worked for you in the past?"

"Codeine," I muttered. "Codeine seems to work best for me. Fifty or sixty milligrams."

"Codeine," he said as he wrote the prescription. "Good. We'll get that right away. Any questions?"

I almost wept.

———

The young doctor left the examination area. While Carrie and I waited for the pharmacy to put together a batch of DDAVP, a nurse I hadn't seen before entered carrying a purple tray full of syringes and test tubes and bags of saline. She sang along faintly with the Muzaked Crosby, Stills, Nash and

Young song that was being piped into the air overhead. She hummed as she read her instructions.

"We need to take some blood, get an IV going, and then we're done," she said. "It'll only take a minute. Make a fist, please." She was one of the many hospital workers who move in and out of your life with breathtaking speed and efficiency, in this instance easing a syringe into a fat vein in my left arm without my feeling so much as a pinch, drawing two test tubes of blood, attaching labels to them, then setting up an IV drip and draping it from a rolling IV pole. Then she picked up her tray and was gone.

Almost immediately the young doctor returned carrying X rays of my ankle. He slipped them into the X-ray reading light. Backlit, they looked like charcoal drawings by Hermann Rorschach.

"There's a fracture of the lateral malleolus," the young doctor said. "Here at the end of the fibula. I compared these X rays with those of your left ankle three months ago. The fractures are nearly identical."

"You're kidding," Carrie said.

"Look," the doctor said, pointing to a tiny sliver of milky light on the X ray. "This fracture is more severe. We won't be able to put a cast on until the bleeding stops and the swelling goes down."

"That happened last time, too," I said.

"This is so weird," Carrie said. "What are the chances of your breaking your right ankle in exactly the same spot as where you broke your left ankle three months ago?"

"Who knows," the doctor said. "Whatever the odds are, you beat them."

"So to speak," I said.

The doctor looked at his watch. "It shouldn't be much —"

My attention drifted. His watch: it had a wide silver elastic-like band. Looking at it made me wonder if the hairs on the top of his wrist ever got caught in the elastic part. The sensation, when a wrist hair was caught in your watchband and plucked out, was a muted echo of the sensation that followed a plucked nose hair. Why was I thinking about this?

"I'm sorry," I said. "Would you repeat what you just said?"

The doctor gave me a surprised look. "I said the DDAVP shouldn't take much longer. Hang in there, okay?"

I nodded, and the doctor left the examination area again.

Carrie held up the overstuffed bag of books she'd been carrying, smiled, and said, "I've got some goodies in here."

Trying not to give evidence of a struggle, I achieved a smile. Carrie reached into the bag and took out two books. The first was *Understanding Horse Psychology,* a textbook for veterinarians. I'd run across the book years ago in the 50¢ bin outside a used-book store. The title and color cover photograph (a lone horse looking positively Freudian as it gazed morosely across a stubble field) hypnotized me, though I hadn't read the book from cover to cover. The other book was titled *A Treasury of the World's Great Letters*. It was an old leathery tome with huge gold letters embossed on the cover and spine. I'd never seen it before.

"There are some other surprises in here, too," Carrie said.

Carrie. She was throwing me a lifeline. And she was throwing it casually, almost imperceptibly, so that I wouldn't feel overwhelmed by it or guilty that I couldn't respond to it.

––––––––––

Often the first dose of codeine takes effect shortly before I am wheeled from the emergency-room examination area to my assigned room in the hospital, a journey that usually involves an elevator ride, so that I have the pleasant sensation of both literal and emotional ascension. So it was on this day. The vigorous elderly man Carrie and I had seen outside the emergency-room entrance, the one who gave us the wheelchair in the first place, wheeled me to my room. I held on to the IV pole, making sure the tubing did not get caught in the wheelchair's wheels as we rolled toward my room. The wheels of the IV stand squeaked loudly and wanted to veer left, like a derelict shopping cart. Carrie walked beside me, carrying the bag of books and her purse.

A nurse joined our caravan as we passed the nurses' station closest to my room. "Hi, I'm Norma," she said. "Let me help you with that." She put a hand on the IV stand, guiding it through the doors as we entered my room. "Hi, George," she said to the elderly volunteer, who smiled and said, "Morning, Norma. Yessir, this one belongs in a museum. Never let me down though." He patted the wheelchair as if it were a well-trained pet.

The room was "semiprivate," meaning it accommodated two patients, though the other bed was empty. I wondered how long I would have the room to myself. Carrie said, "Can we get the bed by the window?" It was unexpectedly moving, that *we*.

"It's all yours," Norma said. Then to George she said, "George, can you give me a hand before you go?"

"Course," the man said. "Happy to."

Together they helped me onto the narrow bed by the window. I looked outside. Snow was falling. It was codeine, breaking up and falling softly over the small field and train tracks, over the plowed roads, over the houses and apartment buildings, the river, the tall trees furred with ice.

I clapped, glancing at the clock every few minutes. Now it was 2:22 P.M. In an hour and eleven minutes it would be 3:33 P.M. An hour and eleven minutes later it would be 4:44 P.M. Numbers. Even their simplest interactions could ricochet in the mind.

More than the world record for clapping, more than a Roberto Clemente baseball card or a Schwinn Sting-Ray (though definitely not more than a Honda XR75, the apotheosis of all my desires), I wanted to discover a new prime number. Why? Did something in me respond to the purity and austerity of numbers, their echoing collisions and reciprocities?

Maybe. But what I remember most was a sense of competition, picked up from my teachers' praise. Praise can ruin you. I would find the newest prime number. Euclid had proved there was no end to them. I made lists of numbers into the millions, looking for primes. I felt guilty about such an ambitious goal. But wouldn't God want me to find a new prime number? After all, hadn't God created the prime numbers in the first place and left them to be discovered like new planets in distant galaxies? On the other hand, you never heard about Jesus doing well in math. . . .

John walked into the dialysis room, stumbling over the edge of the carpet. I laughed.

"*Time wounds all heels*," *I said.*

"*That was funny*," *John said,* "*the first fifty times you said it.*"

PART TWO

Codeine Diary

CODEINE DIARY I

I'm writing this from my bed at the University of Michigan Hospital. It is 3:00 A.M. It is the half-dark of hospitals at night. I have had an accident. I have been in an accident.

From my window I can make out the iced-over Huron River and a tennis court covered with a taut white sheet of snow.

At this point my narrative enters a different order of time.

My goals immediately after my slip on the ice were to find and receive DDAVP and codeine. The elapsed time between my fall and my first dose of codeine was about two hours. My first infusion of DDAVP was administered to me about half an hour later: it took the hospital pharmacy that long to put it together.

The timing was as good as I could hope for — but once the serious pain began, each minute spent waiting for relief felt like a crushed lifetime. For the next week or so, time became alternately turbulent and meditative, depending on how far I was into a dose of codeine. Elastic, elliptical, temperamental, time seemed to spiral out from the center of the bleeding joints. Hospital time only occasionally intersected with chronological time.

I would like to feel a stirring in my knee, calf, and ankle: a signal that the blood pooled there is being absorbed at last and the joints are opening again, like a fist or a jonquil.

Codeine laid its cool hand on my fevered brow. With relief from pain came the urgent desire to pay homage in writing to my surroundings, their sheer *here*-ness, and to pay homage to what was happening to me.

———

There are times, in the last minutes before I am allowed, or allow myself, more codeine, when the pain inside the joints simplifies me utterly. I feel myself descending some sort of evolutionary ladder until I become as crude and guileless as an amoeba. The pain is not personal. I am incidental to it. It is like faith, the believer eclipsed by something immense . . .

———

I wrote the first of these notes in the margins of the January 13 *New York Times*. Above an article about President Bush's nomination of William Bennett as the government's "drug czar," I wrote the words *Codeine Diary*. The *New York Times* does not offer a would-be diarist much of a canvas to work on, and I quickly ran out of room. In the trash can next to my bed I unearthed a couple of relatively clean envelopes and napkins to scribble on (I could lean over just far enough to reach them without upsetting the ice packs on my knee, calf, and ankle), as well as a couple of sheets from a memo pad, at the top of which were printed the words

BR INDUSTRIES, INC. — PRINTERS AND LITHOGRAPHERS
Spanning the Graphic Arts Field

Earlier I noticed the daytime moon. It looked like a nickel that had been run over by a train. It looked like a thumbtack pinned to the blue mat of the sky. No. It looked like a nickel.

I have to watch myself.

Now the pocked and damaged moon is in the window, above a flayed sycamore tree. The sycamore's bark drops to the ground in long curled tongues.

Winter.

Winter. *In this hygienic room, the word arrives from a great distance.*

I am trying to imagine what it feels like outside.

Outside, I imagine, it is so cold that you can feel the air sifting through the hairs in your nostrils.

I would like to feel a stirring.

Here is the window. Here is the sill. Here is the star-tiled floor. Here are the chalk walls. Here is the night-light. Here is the thin table on wheels. Here is the glass of water. Here is the IV pole with its black three-wheeled base. Here are the straps and steel rails on the sides of the bed. Here is the buzzer to the nurses' station. Here is the television in the upper left-hand corner of the room. Here are the urinal and bedpan. Here is the orange vinyl chair. Here are books and magazines Carrie brought me: Understanding Horse Psychology, A Treasury of the World's Great Letters, The Collected Poems of Wallace Stevens, Ordinary Things, From the Hidden Storehouse, Kon-Tiki, Waiting for Godot, Four Plays by Ionesco, The Physical Universe, Motocross Action, Weekly World News, New York Times, The Ultimate Skateboard Book, I & Thou, The Movie Quiz Book, The Oxford Book of Prayer.

The free collision of that list pleases me greatly.

Today is Saturday.

I have had an accident.

I have had an accident on the sidewalk. I watched my feet come out from under me on the iced concrete with a kind of anecdotal perspective. The bleeding inside the joints, the infusions of DDAVP or factor VIII, the weeks of immobility, the waiting for codeine, the inventions with which my mind would veer in the direction of solid ground—as my weight drilled into the twisting leg, I saw the whole pantomime emerge with the clarity of blown glass.

4:00 A.M. It is as quiet as the inside of a brick.

The afternoon soaps started their numbing procession.

John and my mother sat on the brown couch in the dialysis room, intently watching the TV. I sat in John's dialysis chair. Though I stared directly at the TV screen, the images swept vaguely across my eyes. The steady rhythm of clapping urged my mind to drift and twist from my body like a swirl of pipe smoke. I was chasing an idea. I'd never had an idea like this one. It was making me nervous. It could change the world.

What if unknown whole numbers existed in between successive whole numbers but nobody had noticed them? Forget the search for a new prime number. What if between four and six, say, there existed three whole numbers no one knew about, instead of just the one we did know about? Worse, what if the unknown whole numbers existed in a pattern we couldn't predict — two whole numbers between one and two, six whole numbers between two and three, seventy-seven whole numbers between three and four, three between four and five, and on and on? What would happen to our phone number? Our address? Our money in the bank? Everyone's money!

Should I stop clapping and call someone? I tried to explain my theory of unknown whole numbers to John and my mother. John stared at the TV during my explanation. My mother looked confused. She said, "That's good, Tom. Keep using that brain of yours. God gave it to you for a reason."

Without moving his eyes from the TV, with perfect-pitch con-descension, John said, "If you didn't exist, somebody'd have to invent you. Like Alfred Hitchcock."

They both kept watching TV. I struggled to pay attention to the images. Sand sifted through the pinched waist of an hour-glass. A woman wept onto the shoulder of another woman, both kneeling in pouring rain. Two men in three-piece suits glowered at each other across a swanky restaurant.

John was right. My idea was stupid. Obviously.

I did not stop clapping.

THE TEMPTATION TO EXIST

Ellen, the night nurse, walked into my room. It was very early in the morning. She took the ice pack off my right ankle and felt for a pulse where the ice had been. She'd been doing this every five minutes throughout the night to make sure the pressure of bleeding hadn't compressed and finally flattened the blood vessels. If the blood vessels collapsed, the emergency-room doctor had told me, the leg below the knee would have to be amputated. The vigil would last until the morning nurse arrived at 7:00 A.M. If at that time we could find a pulse in the ankle, the risk of amputation would be over.

I was half an hour or so into a dose of codeine: removing the ice pack didn't make me cry out.

"It's still so hot," Ellen said, meaning the skin around the calf. "You could fry an egg on it." She was careful not to disrupt the ice packs on my calf and knee.

I liked Ellen immediately. There is a certain type of ideal nurse I'd been lucky enough to encounter once or twice before. He or she walks a difficult line between no-nonsense meticulousness about the work of nursing and a compassionate and encouraging but absolutely unsentimental bedside manner. The bedside manner of a nurse is even more important than that of a physician, to my mind, though we are not encouraged to think so. For that matter, the nurse *is* a physician: a person skilled in the art of healing. We see and require nurses, and deliver our lives into their capable hands, more frequently than we do hospital doctors at any rate.

Ellen was one of the ideal breed of nurse. She was head-strong, opinionated about every doctor in the hospital, and had a built-in bullshit detector that would put Ernest Hemingway's to shame.

Ellen was a short, round woman in her mid-forties with shoulder-length blond hair. I remember her blue-green eyes. Or rather, I remember noticing that her eyes were blue and green while I tried to figure out what was going on with her contact lenses. The lens edges extended a tad too far into the whites of her eyes. Looking at her, you couldn't help focusing on the edges of her contacts, tiny bluish seams circling the irises like stays of hoopskirts.

"Pulse still there?" I said.

"Yep," Ellen said. "Beating away, just like it's supposed to. How're you feeling?"

"Pretty good, all told," I said. "I was wondering if I could get a notepad of some kind. Something to write on. Anything."

Ellen looked at the various paper products I'd scribbled on and said, "I think we can come up with something. Don't you want to try to get some sleep? You must be tired. You haven't slept a wink since I came on duty."

"I'm going to sleep soon. I just want to write down a few things first."

Ellen leaned over the bed to see what I'd written. She must have thought I was writing a will; she frowned and said, "Don't be silly, Tom. There's no need to worry. You're going to be fine."

"No, no," I said. "It's not a will or anything. I'm just trying to clarify some things. For myself, I mean. I was thinking of writing a poem."

I don't know why I said that last sentence. I had not been thinking of writing a poem — though once I'd said it, I felt an irresistible urge to do so.

"You are?" Ellen's face lifted with interest. "I used to love poetry. Are you a poet?"

I didn't know what to say. It always sounds like a trick question. It's a vastly different question from "Do you write poems?" It seems to mask another question inside it—"Do you consider your own poems to be so good that even though I've never heard of you, you deserve to be called a poet?"

"No," I said. "But I write poems. I mean, I try to."

"I bet you're just being modest," Ellen said. "I've worked with patients who write as a way of coping. I bet poetry's like therapy for you. Oops." She glanced abruptly at her watch. "Sorry. I need to check on something. I'll be back in a second." She hurried out of the room.

I was sorry for the interruption. My most recent dose of codeine had hit full stride, making possible a normal human conversation. Suddenly a conversation seemed the most miraculous and wonderful thing in the world.

Ellen reappeared in less than a minute carrying several pages of typing paper. "Sorry about that," she said. "Here's some paper for you." She sat down on the left edge of the bed, near my healthy foot. "Now, tell me . . . ," she said, "tell me what you write about in your poems. I used to love poetry. I could never write it myself though."

"Who's being modest now?" I said. I was pleased that Ellen felt comfortable enough to sit on the bed.

"I'm not being modest," Ellen said, crossing her legs. "There are things I do well, but poetry's not one of them. Not by a long shot. You're avoiding the question."

"Well," I said, "I've written a lot about my brother. He died of kidney disease in nineteen eighty. We had a dialysis machine in our house, which created a certain, um, rich dynamic in the family. When he died, I experienced a kind of . . . a new kind of self-consciousness. New for me, I mean. It was like having excess consciousness. Poems were a place to put the excess. Make something out of it."

Ellen uncrossed her legs and looked at her watch. "I need to take your ankle's pulse in a minute," she said. "But I don't want you to stop talking."

"No, it's your turn," I said. "I don't want to blabber on."

"Oh, I'll have my turn all right," Ellen said. "Don't worry about that. When I get going, you can't shut me up. I want to know about your poems. Is writing like therapy for you?"

I looked at the floor. "Actually, I was hoping the topic of poetry-as-therapy wouldn't come up again."

"Why's that?" Ellen asked.

"I don't know how committed you are to the idea. This is the first conversation I've had in a while that isn't about pain or bleeding, and I don't want to blow it."

Ellen shrugged her shoulders. "Just tell me what you think," she said. "You don't need to pussyfoot around me."

"Okay," I said, grinning. "No pussyfooting. Well, I think that . . . that *writing* is therapeutic, but poetry is something you *make* out of your writing. Making a poem is probably therapeutic in the way that gardening is, or painting is, or learning to shoot a jump shot is. By requiring powers of concentration and attention that you didn't know you had in you."

"What could be more therapeutic than that?" Ellen asked.

"Exactly," I said. "But you can't count on it. Most of the time you're just working in the dark trying to find a pattern that will unlock meaning — or unlock the process of making meaning. God, I don't mean to sound so academic."

Ellen shook her head. "What did I just tell you? Say what you think and stop apologizing. You're like my daughter Mary Jo, she's always apologizing. Mind you, she's done things."

"She has?" I said, sensing Ellen wanted to talk about her daughter. "Good—here's my chance to change the subject." I tried to lean forward a bit to show Ellen I was interested. "Tell me about your daughter. I mean, if you want to."

"Is this the time to go into it?" Ellen whispered, and I wasn't sure if she spoke to herself or to me. To be safe, I replied: "It is if you like."

Ellen turned her head to the window and stared outside. The river, the tennis court, black night. Ellen sighed. Her sigh seemed to release an unutterable sadness into the room.

"My little one," Ellen said, "Mary Jo, she's engaged to this fellow Dave." She winced.

I tried to look sympathetic. "He's bad news?"

"He's got Mary Jo into drugs. Walk into his house, there's his drug paraphernalia in the corner of the living room. First thing you see."

"You've been to his house," I said incredulously, "and he left all that stuff where you could see it? He didn't even throw it into a closet?"

"That's right," Ellen said. "He said it was his friend's. But Mary Jo doesn't lie to me. Mary Jo, she and I have the kind of relationship where we tell each other everything."

"Wow. I bet that's a mixed blessing," I said.

"It causes me all kinds of grief, but I wouldn't want it any other way. I figured the truth would always be better than my suspicions. I said to her, 'Tell me the truth no matter how much you think it'll upset me.' Once I said that, I had to learn to take my medicine. She told me how Dave buys his syringes from this old diabetic woman who lives down the street. The woman gets more than she needs and sells the rest. Makes a pretty profit. She probably supplies all of Michigan with syringes."

Ellen paused to look at her watch, then continued. "Dave has her freebasing cocaine. Mary Jo says he puts it in ammonia to separate the paste out so he can smoke it. He cuts it with vitamin B or baby laxative. It makes me — "

"Baby laxative?" I interrupted. I was dizzied by the specificity of information Ellen was giving me.

"That's right. I tell you, that man is a piece of work. Mary Jo told me they were engaged, and then she said Dave accidentally asked his father *and* a friend to be the best man. Both of them! Said he had to straighten it out. 'I guess he does!' I said to Mary Jo."

Ellen's face fired; she squinted her eyes.

"We don't have to talk about this," I said, "if you don't want to."

"You're kind," Ellen said. She took a deep breath. "He gets me upset. He was brought up by this wealthy family, but he just buys drugs with the money they send him. That boy had braces for eight years! Then he got stoned at a concert and fell flat on his jaw. Ruined his teeth. All that dental work down the drain. His jaw was wired together; he was in the hospital for a month. What did he do? He melted his morphine down so he and his buddies and my Mary Jo could inject it. Right there in the hospital!"

"*This* hospital?" I asked.

"No," Ellen said. "I don't know what I'd do if he came here. Probably have somebody watch him twenty-four hours a day."

"Like what you're having to do with me," I said. The ice in the ice pack on my ankle shifted, and the pack fell off onto the bed. Ellen picked it up. Most of the ice had melted. Ellen took the ice packs off my knee and calf as well and stood up. "I'll get you some more ice," she said, walking toward the door. "You need a break from my gabbing. Want anything besides ice?"

"No thanks," I said.

I was gorging on conversation. Ellen couldn't talk long enough for me. I wanted to know all about Mary Jo and Dave and about Ellen herself. In the back of my mind, though, the urge to work on a poem competed for my attention. On a sheet from the BR Industries, Inc. memo pad (I wanted to save the typing paper for later), I wrote three lines:

The chalk walls through the long night

The chalk walls through the night hours

The chalk walls through the listening night

Earlier I had written a sentence — "Here are the chalk walls" — the sounds of which had been nudging my ear all through my conversation with Ellen. Auditioning the words *chalk walls* in these three lines made me pessimistic about being able to use them in a poem. I liked the slowness of the sound, but all three lines were finally too sonorous; they tried too hard to "climb the stiles of English influence," a phrase Louis Zukofsky used to criticize a Wallace Stevens poem. Could I surround the line with others that would turn down the stile-climbing volume?

Ellen entered the room carrying fresh ice packs. When she saw me scribbling, she started laughing and said, "You're writing down everything I told you! Blackmailer!"

I laughed, too. I said, "My instructions will be very precise. Small unmarked bills will be fine. Or large marked ones. Whichever."

Chuckling, Ellen felt for a pulse in my right ankle before positioning the new ice pack. She took care that the edges of the fresh ice cubes did not dig into the bleed. "That's great," I said. "Thanks."

"Good," Ellen said, looking at my ankle. "You're kind to listen to my gabbing."

"There's no kindness involved," I said. "We're just getting warmed up."

"Are you sure you don't want to sleep?" Ellen said. "I should let you sleep."

"No, no," I said. "Let's talk some more. I mean, if you can."

"Let me check on one last thing," Ellen said. "Then we can talk till we're blue in the face."

"That's what I want," I said. "Blue faces. We need blue faces around here." Ellen winked and walked out the door.

As soon as she was gone, I looked at the three lines I'd written. Below them I wrote a three-line stanza:

Your second breath says it, and the room's tick,
the star-tiled floor,
the chalk walls through the night hours . . .

The first draft of a poem was ahead in the distance, coming into view. Immediately my leg felt better. That sounds ridiculous, and yet it's true. It was impossible for me to spend any time at all in a hospital and not think almost constantly of John. John was clearly the *you* of this stanza. Integrating his continual presence into language lessened the weight of him somehow. The poet Charles Wright once said that he wrote poems to "summon the spirits up and set the body to music." Summoning John in a poem acquitted my leg (I know this sounds preposterous) of the burden of John's previous hospital stays. And in an equally inexplicable way, piecing together a stanza that pleased my ear introduced rhythm to my body. Why did I resist affirming that writing a poem was therapeutic? Who was I kidding?

We're headed in the right direction, I thought as I read the stanza over and over. *Chalk walls* didn't stand out the way I'd feared it would. But what was the *it* that "your second breath says"? Death? Sleep? Insomnia? Alertness? I didn't know, and at that point I didn't need to know. I thought of Charles Simic, another favorite poet, who said that *it* was the most interesting word in the English language.

"Want to read it to me?" Ellen said, and I flinched instantly. I hadn't seen her enter the room. I had no idea how long she'd been standing there watching me.

"You scared the crap out of me," I said.

"You're in the right place then," Ellen joked. "We can handle any bowel-related emergency."

We both laughed.

Talking with Ellen, I was actually happy. Safely ensconced within a dose of codeine, I had a hunger for humor and companionship and conversation, even a capacity for happiness. As soon as the codeine wore off, I felt separated from other people as though by a thick veneer of hard wax. I couldn't stand the thought of anyone's company besides Carrie's, and I could hardly speak.

"Why don't you read it to me?" Ellen said, pointing to the stanza I'd written. "I'd love to hear it."

"Oh, no," I said. "I don't know what I've got here. It's too early to read it out loud."

"Okay," Ellen said. "But when it's done, I want to hear it."

"That's a deal," I said. "Meantime, get cracking on those marked bills."

"Oh, *I* see," Ellen said, sitting down again on the left side of the bed. "You're a wolf in sheep's clothing. You've got that innocent clean-cut look, but it doesn't fool me. Not for a — Oh! Sorry!"

The bed shook as Ellen sat down, jostling my right leg slightly. I grimaced, expecting a stab of pain that never came. Ellen stood up immediately. She looked mortified.

"It's okay," I said. "No harm done."

"Some nurse!" Ellen said.

"It's really okay," I said. "I swear. You can sit down."

Ellen sat down with exaggerated care. I was tempted to howl with faked pain as soon as she touched the bed, but I decided not to cry wolf.

"You're really okay?" Ellen said.

"I am," I said. "I swear."

"All right then," Ellen said, putting the incident behind us and settling in for a long talk. "What should we talk about?"

————————

Our marathon discussion lasted until about six in the morning. I, or my leg, was pretty much the extent of Ellen's duties that night. Sometimes she left the room after taking my leg's pulse, but usually she stayed and talked, since she'd have to be back in five minutes anyway. There were moments of silence when it appeared our conversation had run its course; we found ourselves in an awkward postinebriated state, hungover from so much mutual self-disclosure, shy with our new knowledge of each other. But then one of us would ask a question or make an observation, and we were off again. Hair of the dog.

"Nixon's problem is, he's not eating right," my mother said. "It's plain as day; anyone can see it. Just look at the man."

It was 5:30 P.M. and I was still at it, 120 claps per minute.

My father, just home from work, walked into the kitchen to say hello to my mother and me. Surveying the scene, he set his briefcase on the kitchen counter and said to himself, "Care for a drink? Don't mind if I do, thank you for asking."

WAYS OF ESCAPE

They have been at a great feast of languages, and stolen the scraps.

— Shakespeare

I must have dozed off for at least a few minutes that first night in the hospital. I woke during a dream I'd had many times as a child.

John and I were in the dialysis room in our house in Charleston. Outside, night fell over the stilled houses and potholed driveways of our street. Stars flashed and hung. John was dialyzing, the machine running smoothly, his bright blood shuttling through the lattice of tubing. I stared at the machine: the water pump, the coils, the subtle positioning of the scissor clamps. I was nervous. It had been hours since my mother and father had gone somewhere on an errand, and I was afraid something would go wrong with the machine.

John pulled at his beard. Dialysis seemed to suck the light from his face. Inspecting the shunt, he said, "We have to redress it now."

I stared at the shunt, a straw-sized tube impaling the flesh above the inside of his wrist. The shunt shamed and silenced me. His blood left his body and returned through the shunt. I'd seen my parents re-dress it. The process looked complex and difficult.

"We'd better wait," I said.

"For what?" John asked.

"Mom or Dad."

"They've gone."

"Where?"

John said nothing. He gave me a sphinxlike grin.

What followed occurred in the slow motion of great clarity. John and I collaborated like renal specialists. With scissor clamps I cut off the blood's flow to and from the shunt. Alarms bleeped like telephones. I helped John unwrap the gauze around the shunt, and together we removed the plastic tube from his wrist as though it were a simple IV needle. The tube was empty now but speckled with wet blood. John stood up. His legs were unstable, his having sat in the dialysis chair for more than six hours, but he quickly caught his balance. He gestured for me to sit down.

"Your turn," John said.

I sat down and rolled up my sleeve.

It was a sudden sensation of flight, watching my blood travel from the shunt above my wrist into the lattice of tubing, through the coils and back again, in time, into my arm. John said my own kidneys would soon shrink, obsolete, to the size of chestnuts. We talked about the possibility of a transplant: he would contact a nephrologist at the Cleveland Clinic to get my name on a waiting list—

———

I felt a hand on my ankle. "Sorry," Ellen said. "I was hoping I wouldn't wake you up. Go back to sleep."

"No," I said, groggily, "I don't think I want that. I want to be awake. Can we talk? God, I sound like Joan Rivers."

"I've always liked her," Ellen said. "She's so brassy. She never hides her plastic surgeries. She's always out in the open with them."

Feeling more alert, I said, "I'll always respect her for directing and being in absolutely the worst movie ever made."

"What was that?"

"*Rabbit Test.* About a man who gets pregnant. A close second has to be *Gas,* starring Donald Sutherland. It was about the gasoline crisis. I can't believe I fell asleep. I must've cut you off mid-sentence."

"Yes, well, I've gotten over it," Ellen said, sighing deeply, imitating bitter disappointment. "After my divorce and three ungrateful kids, it was only a minor blow to the ego."

"Give me a break," I said, pretending to play an invisible violin. "Maybe I should go back to sleep."

"Watch it, smart-ass," Ellen said. "Don't forget, I'm the one with the codeine."

———

In *Ways of Escape,* the second volume of his autobiography, Graham Greene wrote, "I can see now that my travels, as much as the act of writing, were ways of escape," and quoted Auden: "Man needs escape as he needs food and deep sleep." To spend any time at all in a hospital is to recognize the fierceness of that truth. Throughout the first night following my fall on the ice, my conversations with Ellen, subsidized by codeine, were escapes of the first order. Conversation was to me what travel was to Greene. What follows are table scraps left over from the feast — the few I can remember or that I jotted down in my notebook.

———

Ellen said, "My husband used to feed his dog gunpowder to make it mean to strangers. It worked."

———

Ellen said, "When I was a girl, we had a baby deer. Daddy brought her home in his hard hat. I named her Ninny. She sounded just like a baby sheep. You had to wear shoes when you fed her with a milk bottle. She'd step on your feet trying to get closer to the bottle. Milk'd be dripping down her throat and all over your feet. I had white spots on my shoes for a year."

———

I said, "My mother told me that every time I lied, I put another thorn in Jesus' head."

———

I said, "It's strange how little racing there was in motocross. I mean actual racing—where you get in a dogfight over a position. Usually we settled into our places early in the motos, as if they'd been determined by God. Now that I think about it, the race was probably over during practice. We went out and after a few laps decided who was faster than us and who we were faster than. And sure enough, that's how the race would turn out."

"You were a bunch of . . . what's the word . . . *Calvinist* dirt-bikers," Ellen said.

"Now that," I said, "is hitting below the belt."

———

"Do you have kids?" Ellen said.

"No," I said.

"Does having hemophilia make you not want to have any?"

"Yeah, I think so. If we had a son, he'd be fine. But if we had a daughter, she'd be a carrier. For some reason, I always thought that if Carrie and I had a child, it'd be a girl. You never know, though. By the time our daughter—if we had a daughter—by the time *she* had children, maybe there'd be all sorts of medical breakthroughs."

"Oh, you can count on that," Ellen said. "It's amazing what they're doing."

"The thing that sounds great to me is the liver patch. Have you heard anything about that one?" Ellen shook her head. "It's like a smoker's patch that would release factor VIII right into the liver."

"That *would* be great," Ellen said.

"Then again," I said, "you can't count on medical breakthroughs. And anyway, do I want to put a kid through having hemophilia?"

"But you're talking two generations down the road. You *know* they're going to come up with incredible things by then."

"I hope so. I think so. That's when I wonder if I'm just using hemophilia as an excuse. I know I don't want kids, but maybe that's just because the idea terrifies me."

"That's good. That's smart. Terror of kids is good."

Ellen: "I think men just hang around me till they get the hang of life again. They lean on me till they get the swing of life back."

Ellen: "Mary Jo says Dave gets an ounce for forty-one dollars and sells it for sixty-five. Says he could sell it for seventy-five, but he likes to give people a bargain."

"Tom, you awake?"

"Yes."

"How you feeling?"

"Pretty good. I wish I could move around. Take a shower or something."

"Want me to get you a washcloth?"

"No thanks. I'm too comfortable to move. I don't want to risk losing this position."

"Let me ask you something, Tom. Do you believe in God?"

"Well, the short answer is yes, and the long answer is yes. What about you?"

"Me? I used to. I mean, I want to be a good person and all. But I don't see how a God can let everything that happens happen. I think working in a hospital either makes your faith stronger or squashes it like a fly."

"Oh, there was a time when I thought *everything* was about hemophilia," I said. "The secret agenda of punk was hemophilia. Same with motocross, skateboarding. Christianity."

"Christianity? How'd you figure that one?"

"It was all about hemophilia. The blood of the lamb. Take this blood which is shed for thee. All that. I figured Jesus was a very well-adjusted chronic bleeder."

"I did read that book [Bernie Siegel's *Love, Medicine and Miracles*]," Ellen said. "And there was a hemophiliac here once whose mind and body were definitely tuned in to the same frequency. All he had to do was look at a bottle of aspirin and he'd start a bleed."

"The Clash and the Gang of Four are my bands," I said. "And Elvis Costello. The Fastbacks. The Raincoats."

"I can't *stand* that kind of music," Ellen said. "Johnny Rotten? *Yuck*. Don't even talk about it. I don't want to hear it. Next topic."

I said, "Would it be all right if I switched beds? Before I get a roommate?"

"We usually can't do that," Ellen said. "I thought you wanted the window?"

"I did. But I want to be able to hear voices better. I asked one of my poetry professors once if he ever considered writing plays, and he said he wasn't interested enough in people. I want to hear people's voices better. I want to be more interested in people."

"I'll see what I can do. You're getting a roommmate in the morning. His paperwork . . . just don't get your hopes up."

"I told you," Ellen said. "I'm hopeless. Just the thought of a math test makes my stomach tense up."

"Okay, wait. Don't give up yet. We're not talking about taking a test. We're just talking about the way mathematicians see things. Here's an example, the best example I know. There was this German mathematician named Carl Friedrich Gauss. Most mathematicians I know say he was the best who ever lived. When Gauss was a kid in school, his teacher asked the class to add up all the numbers between one and a hundred. The teacher probably thought he was giving himself a ten-minute break or something. Gauss had the answer in a few seconds. He saw that one plus a hundred is a hundred and one, two plus ninety-nine is a hundred and one, three plus ninety-eight is a hundred and one, and so on. He saw that there were fifty pairs of numbers that added up to a hundred and one. The answer had to be fifty times a hundred and one, which is five thousand fifty. See what I mean? The point is he saw a *pattern* in the numbers that *had* to lead to the answer. He didn't have to add up all those numbers."

"I can see that," Ellen said. "I can. But it doesn't do anything for me. It's like watching figure skating on TV. It's great that there are people who can do all those flips and spins and stuff. But I'm sure as hell not going to go out and do it myself."

"Tell me about it!" I said.

"Tell you nothing. You're problem is, you *would* go out and do it."

———

The codeine had worn off. I tried to remain as still as possible. The skin was boiling, sharp dots of heat along the leg like water bubbling in a pan. Or, alternately, an even heat just under the skin's surface, a steady flaming intensity.

"You're doing great, Tom," Ellen said. "It's almost seven. Your leg's going to be fine. You're going to be fine."

From the 1971 Guinness Book of World Records:

Clapping. The duration record for continuous clapping is 14 hours 6 minutes by Nicolas Willey, 18, and Christopher Floyd, 17, of Canford School, Dorset, England, on December 13-14, 1968. They sustained an average of 140 claps per minute and an audibility range of at least 100 yards.

EMILY DICKINSON, ANGIE DICKINSON, ECSTASY, ETC.

Because the weight of the bedsheet and blanket across my flushed leg was too great, I asked Carrie to bring to the hospital a prop I'd made years earlier out of an old cardboard box. I'd cut off its top and bottom, as well as one of the four sides. The result was a kind of bridge supporting the sheet and blanket, under which the leg lay like a limestone deposit.

Carrie sat in the orange vinyl chair beside my bed, reading *A Treasury of the World's Great Letters*.

"Want to hear any of these letters?" Carrie asked. Her eyes moved up and down the table of contents. "'Alexander the Great and King Darius the Third Exchange Defiance for the Mastery of the World.' Sound juicy?"

"What are some others?" I said absently, fingering the bedsheet.

"Let's see," she said. "'Agrippina, Nero's Mother, Pleads to Her Emperor-Son for Her Own Life,' 'Emily Dickinson Finds Ecstasy in the Mere Sense of Living,' 'William James Discovers That He Has Omitted the Deepest Principle of Human Nature from His Textbook on Psychology.'"

"Where'd you get that?" I interrupted, taking an interest.

"I think I picked it up at your parents' house. The last time we were there. There's a stamp on the title page—TRINITY METHODIST CHURCH LIBRARY, GRAND RAPIDS, MICHIGAN. Look at this," she said, holding the book up so I could see the title page, "it's got one of those old-fashioned superlong subtitles you like."

"All right!" I said. "Read the whole thing. Don't leave me hanging."

Carrie stiffened her posture and dropped the corners of her mouth, feigning pretentious self-regard and an English accent. "Ahem. Yes, in case you were wondering, I am an Anglophile. Indubitably."

"You sound like a cross between William F. Buckley and Lady Di," I said.

"Please, young man," Carrie said, scolding me in character. "The full title of the book is as follows: *A Treasury of the World's Great Letters: From Ancient Days to Our Own Time, Containing the Characteristic and Crucial Communications, and Intimate Exchanges and Cycles of Correspondence, of Many of the Outstanding Figures of World History, and Some Notable Contemporaries, Selected, Edited, and Integrated with Biographical Backgrounds and Historical Settings and Consequences,* by M. Lincoln Schuster. Whew."

"Wow. That Mr. Schuster, he was one modest guy," I said. "But I do love long subtitles. It's like saying that the title — the first title, the title before the colon — can't possibly embody the richness and variety of the world. It's like saying to the reader, 'Reader, the world is bigger than my book. The world dumbfounds me. But maybe a subtitle can hint at how rich and strange it is.' What made you pick it up anyway?"

My dissertation on subtitles exhausted Carrie's Anglophilia; she returned to herself. "Oh, I don't know," she said. "I guess I wanted to take a break from *Tom Jones*."

We both chuckled. Carrie had been reading *Tom Jones* on and off for two years, in between books on graphic design and journals like *Print* and *Graphis,* and she was hilariously (and needlessly) self-deprecating about it.

"Don't you, like, want to know," Carrie continued, suddenly imitating valley girl speech as she looked again at the table of contents, "how Emily Dickinson found, like, ecstasy in the mere sense of, gag me with a spoon, living?"

"I do, I do," I said, laughing.

Carrie flipped through the book looking for Emily Dickinson's letter. When she found it she said, "*Oh. My. God.* I'm like, soooo excited!"

After we both calmed down a bit, Carrie admonished herself, "Okay, Carrie, you can stop that now," her lovely Midwestern lilt (a phrase that until I met Carrie, I might have judged an oxymoron) returning to her voice again. "Here we go. 'August nineteen seventy'—I mean eighteen seventy. 'August eighteen seventy. Truth is such a rare thing, it is delightful to tell it. I find ecstasy in living.' This is Emily Dickinson's letter, by the way. Did I make that clear?"

"I *was* a little confused," I said, smiling. "Thanks for clarifying."

"No problem," Carrie said. "Where was I?"

"'I find ecstasy in living,'" I said.

"Is *everything* about *you?*" Carrie joked, her eyes dancing joyously. "Okay. Here we go. I know, I already said that." She startled to giggle, abruptly fought the impulse, held her breath as if to suppress hiccups, then broke out into helpless laughter. I joined in with a crescendo of my own.

Laughter echoed through the small room. For a minute or two we were elsewhere, given a reprieve from the grim hospital. I forgot entirely about my leg. Codeine made this reprieve physically possible, but Carrie made it a psychological reality. Chemicals took away the pain and left me acutely aware of the antiseptic, anonymous room. Carrie's generosity of spirit urged my mind out of the hospital altogether.

Carrie took a deep breath. "Okay, Carrie," she repeated. "Just read the letter by Emily Dickinson. 'I find — '"

I couldn't help myself. "Emily Dickinson. Wasn't she in that TV show about the policewoman? *Killer Cop, Mrs. Kojak,* something like that? Wait — maybe it was just called *Police Woman?*"

"That's *Angie* Dickinson. This is Emily Dickinson, Angie Dickinson's great-great-great-grandmother."

"Oh. I see," I said, acting relieved. "Thanks again for clarifying."

Carrie wore a manic grin. "Do you want to hear the fucking letter or not?"

"Yes," I said. "Please. I'll be good."

We were able to stop laughing but couldn't erase the grins from our faces. Carrie began again. "'I find ecstasy in living; the mere sense of living is joy enough. How do most people live without any thoughts? There are many people in the world — you must have noticed them in the street — how do they live? How do they get the strength to put on their clothes in the morning?'"

Emily Dickinson's letter was so at odds with the antic spirit of the room that I asked Carrie to read it again.

This time her voice did not betray any hint of our high jinks. "'Truth is such a rare thing, it is delightful to tell it. I find ecstasy in living; the mere sense of living is joy enough. How do most people live without any thoughts? There are many people in the world — you must have noticed them in the street — how do they live? How do they get the strength to put on their clothes in the morning?'"

A long silence.

"Maybe," Carrie said at last, "we should switch to *Understanding Horse Psychology.*"

So: *the current world record for clapping was held by two English teenagers. I didn't understand. Why did it take two people?* Did the *Guinness Book people require more than one clapper, or had the two teenagers simply decided to share the glory? Did they clap in unison, or take turns? Had I misunderstood the whole concept of clapping? Surely Nicolas Willey and Christopher Floyd had not played patty-cake for fourteen hours and six minutes?*

I thought of writing them a letter.

September 7, 1972

Nicolas Willey and Christopher Floyd
Canford School
Dorset
England

Dear Nicolas Willey and Christopher Floyd,

I am eleven years old and I want to ask you a few questions about your world record for clapping. Why did it take two people? Did you both clap the whole time? Did you take turns?

How did you decide to break the record? I have decided either to cook more than 75 omelettes in half an hour or clap longer than 14 hours and 6 minutes, your record. I think I am going to clap. I hope there will be no hard feelings.

> *Sincerely,*
> *Tom Andrews*

In the end I decided against the letter. It might have given the two teenagers the idea to break their own record before I had a chance at it.

SUNDAY MORNING

My roommate, an elderly man with end-stage heart disease, was rolled into the room on a stretcher. Oxygen tubes curled around his ears, lined his cheek, entered his nostrils. His wife read newspapers while he slept. They looked uncannily alike: white-haired, slight, their salmon-colored faces stretched tightly across the facial bones.

Sometimes his breathing sped up suddenly, like quick deep hits on a cigarette. This lasted only a few seconds.

Hours passed. He had yet to be awake in our room. His lungs labored through sleep, each breath a furrow plowed in earth.

About nine o'clock in the evening, after Carrie went home and I'd spent an hour or so writing in a notebook she'd brought me, I drifted off to sleep myself. When I woke, my roommate was watching *The Tonight Show*. Johnny Carson's guest was Blair Brown.

"Sure, I like redheads," Johnny Carson said. "I have friends who are redheads."

I looked over at my roommate. He looked surprisingly alert. His wife continued to read newspapers. A commercial interrupted *The Tonight Show,* and my roommate caught me looking at him. He smiled at me. He had the kind of horsey smile whereby his upper lip rose well above the gumline. His exposed gums described the shape of each tooth's root, like Saran Wrap over brass knuckles.

"My name is Leonard," he said. "Enid here—this is my wife, Enid."

Enid smiled at me. She stood up to adjust the pillow behind Leonard's back, but he shook his head and hands and she sat down.

"I'm Tom," I said. I wondered if I should say, "Pleased to meet you," followed by "I wish we could have met under different circumstances" or something else.

Before I could make a decision, Leonard said, "Are you married, Tom?"

Enid sat back down in the yellow vinyl chair beside Leonard's bed—identical to the orange one beside my bed—and opened a newspaper.

"Yes. I am," I said. "I've been married for four years now." I sounded like I was trying to convince him. "That was Carrie with me this afternoon."

"That's good," Leonard said, still smiling. "It's good to have somebody with you, isn't it?" His smile was too severe, as though the taut skin of his face needed to be stretched out before the workout of conversation.

"Yes," I said. "It is."

Enid rustled her newspaper.

Leonard pointed to the notebook on my lap and said, "You a writer?"

I swallowed. "Me? No. I work as an editor for a mathematics journal. Well, a copyeditor."

"Hear that, Enid? He's got that calculus in him. I could tell by looking at him, he's got that calculus in him."

Leonard laughed—at least, I think it was laughter. His laugh was a cross between snorting and coughing. I worried about the tubes in his nostrils as laughter jerked his head.

"Easy, honey," Enid said without looking up from her newspaper.

Leonard quieted enough to ask, "What are you working on there?"

"I'm not sure, really," I said. "I've been trying to write a poem. I was making a list of words I might use. Sounds ridiculous, I know."

I looked at the list I'd started, the beginning of a word-hoard: *long, knot, dissolve (as noun), quartz, paper cup.*

"List of words. Uh-huh," Leonard said. "I tell you, somebody ought to write a book about my life. Sell it to the movies. It'd be better than a miniseries. You want to write it? You could write it up."

"Um . . . "

The eruptive painful sound of his laughter.

Tuesday Morning

Hi Tom!

Congratulations! You must have won your "endurance test" (in clapping) with flying colors. Buddy sent clippings from the paper to Vada — then too I had a good phone talk with Uncle Okey yesterday morning. So glad everyone had a Happy Thanksgiving.

Hope John gets his fruit I had sent from Sears soon and it isn't spoiled or too green. Drop me a card and kiss mother for me.

Love — Aunt Betty

CODEINE DIARY II

My leg shimmers, spreading its colors like a peacock: cinnabar, copper, rust, olive, ruddle, gentian violet, umber . . .

––––––

The German poet Günter Eich wrote that "In each good line of poetry I hear the cane of the blindman striking: I am on secure ground now." Good or bad, each sentence I get down before the codeine wears off is a toehold toward equilibrium. Each phrase, quotation, memory.

––––––

A girl and a boy in the hallway outside our door.
GIRL: I can move my eyes in different directions.
BOY: I can pull my eyes out like cue balls.
GIRL: Cannot!

––––––

It's dislocating, not having an appetite for days. Not desiring sex. At times not even desiring an end to pain. To lie awake at night utterly without desire. William Blake's cry— "I want! I want!"—is like a bewildering voice from an inverse world.

––––––

Arterial sunrise, capillary dusk.

––––––

When I told my first hematologist that I had raced motocross, that in fact in one race in Gallipolis, Ohio, I had gotten the holeshot and was bumped in the first turn and run over by twenty-some motorcycles, she said, "No. Not with your factor level. I'm sorry, but you wouldn't withstand the head injuries. You like the sound of yourself being dramatic."

———————

Heels clicking by in the hallway.

———————

Desirelessness. It does not, surprisingly, lead to suicidal fantasies. Those *fantasies arrive with images of almost unlimited desire: to be gone, to erase myself from the created world. They are anti-urges, yes, but they are as ferocious and consuming as thirst to the dehydrated.*

Thinking of suicide means imagining myself without desire at the precise moment when I am most full of desire. But if I'm successful in imagining that, then I no longer desire to kill myself.

———————

You like the sound of yourself being dramatic.

———————

There is a sleep like the ~~broad~~ dissolve

There is a sleep like the long dissolve
You are never tired enough

Sometimes the carapace of cliché that enshrouds the imagination seems impenetrable. I keep thinking of P. G. Wodehouse's spoof of poets who write phrases like "pale parabola of joy." Is it possible to chip away enough of the carapace to let

some wildness or unpredictability or something — *anything* —
*into the poem? Maybe painting would be better. Carrie, with
face. John, with arm. Dialysis machine, with cloud cover and
fireweed in a junkyard: rusted Buicks and old bathtubs lodged
in the landscape . . .*

———

Sunrise. The sky gray and pink.

———

This fierce inward stalking of patience.

"You have to imagine Richard Nixon as a little boy," my mother said. "A boy with a mother and father, just like everybody else."

Now I tried to muffle the sound of my clapping.

"It's not that simple," my father said, "and you know it."

THE PILGRIM'S REGRESS

*To glimpse the essential. . . . Stay flat on your
back all day long, and moan. . . .*
— E. M. CIORAN

I spoke in between moans. I said, "What do you think she meant by 'without any thoughts'? That people don't have thoughts, or that they don't have *serious* thoughts?"

Carrie looked up from *Tom Jones*. She said, "What's that? Who?"

"Emily Dickinson," I said. "Do you think she really meant that people don't have *any* thoughts? I mean, how could she know?"

"You're still thinking about that letter I read you?"

"I keep thinking about her question, 'How do most people live without any thoughts?' Do you think she meant 'How do most people live without any *serious* thoughts?' Wouldn't a better question be 'How do most people live *with* thoughts?' She seems astonished that people who don't have thoughts — or serious thoughts, I guess — can gather up the strength to put their clothes on. But don't serious thoughts hurt your chances of putting your clothes on more than they help?"

"You feel that way now. But I bet you'll change your mind when your painkillers come. Or at least when you get out of here, when you can get on your feet. Your thoughts are pursuing you, I can see that. They're making you question everything you hold sacred. Even Emily Dickinson."

The Holy Spirit was nice, but the Holy Ghost was scary.

Jesus was the Son. Jesus was a real person, and Jesus was God, too. God was only God, but Jesus was God and a real person.

God was the Father. He saw it all. He saw everything. He was inside your heart, inside the place where you made decisions.

God watched jealously while I clapped my hands without thinking of Him.

Jealously, He watched.

VARIATIONS, CALYPSO, AND FUGUE ON A THEME OF JOHN ASHBERY

66 I have a surprise," Carrie said.

Carrie pulled from behind her back two copies of *As We Know,* a book of poems by John Ashbery, and insisted that we read, together, "Litany," a poem for two voices to be read simultaneously. On each page of the poem are two thin columns of words. "You read the right column," Carrie said, handing me one of the books. "It'll be fun. The poem's seventy pages long, but let's just read a couple of pages to see how it goes. Okay? On three."

"Hold on," I said, thumbing through the book to find the first page of "Litany."

Carrie waited until I was ready, cleared her throat, and said, "One, two, three — "

For someone like me	*So this must be a hole*
The simplest things	*Of cloud —*
Like having toast or —	

"Wait a second," I interrupted. "I screwed up *cloud*. I think I said *crowd*."

"Don't worry," Carrie said. "You can't mess it up. Just relax."

"Okay," I said. "I'm relaxed."

Carrie said, "One, two, three — "

Going to church are	*So this must be a hole*
Kept in one place —	*Of cloud —*

"I'm sorry," I said, interrupting again. "I thought we were starting over. My mistake."

"*Fine,*" Carrie said, holding back a minor ripple of impatience. "We'll start over. Ready? One, two, three — "

For someone like me	*So this must be a hole*
The simplest things	*Of cloud*
Like having toast or	*Mandate or trap*
Going to church are	*But haze that casts*
Kept in one place . . .	*The milk of enchantment . . .*

We started slowly, cautiously. Soon we felt like Zoot Sims and Stan Getz, listening hard to each other until we stumbled onto a rhythm and a tone that welcomed us into the poem even though we didn't understand it, we didn't have a clue. Our voices fused, broke off, meandered, hesitated, fused again, broke off again. We were exhilarated, caught off guard by exhilaration. What were we making together here? Whatever it was, its delicious incarnation lasted only as long as we kept going.

We read for about ten minutes, in the end giddy and fumbling over words, when Susan, one of the afternoon nurses, walked in.

"What in the world are you guys doing?" Susan asked.

Carrie and I just looked at each other, wondering where to begin.

My mother asked Mrs. Flowers to come over and watch me for a while. The Flowerses lived near the public swimming pool on Parkwood Road. To get to Parkwood Road, you took Smith Road, which rose and fell and sliced through a series of steep hills. Riding your bike on Smith Road was like riding a motocross track, or what I imagined a motocross track to be like. You could haul ass down the hill by the Schultzes' house and catch air — well, a little bit, if you timed your launch right — at the sudden rise by the Vogelbachs'.

Mrs. Flowers said okay. She would stop by in the afternoon to be a witness to my world record attempt; later she would sign an affidavit if we needed her to. Hearing my mother's half of the phone conversation made me cringe.

"Ellie, I don't know how to ask you this," my mother said. "Tom's . . . Tom's clapping . . . Tom got the Guinness Book of World Records for his birthday last year, and he hasn't put it down since. He's got it in his mind to break a world record and get in that book. He wanted to cook more than seventy-five omelettes in half an hour or clap his hands for longer than fourteen hours."

Mrs. Flowers said something that made my mother laugh.

"Right, Ellie," my mother said. "I told him, 'Not in my kitchen you're not!' So he decided to clap his hands, and he's right here beside me clapping."

Again Mrs. Flowers said something that made my mother laugh.

"No," my mother said. "Somehow I don't get the idea he's applauding me."

————————

Mrs. Flowers and my mother sat on the blue-and-white couch in the living room and talked while I clapped and clapped, perched on the piano bench.

"Tom," Mrs. Flowers said at one point, "why do you want to be in the Guinness Book of World Records?"

No one had asked me that before. I wasn't sure what to say. I stalled for time by standing up and walking to a chair closer to Mrs. Flowers. My mother was watching me very closely.

"For God," I lied for the second time that day, looking at my shoes.

Mrs. Flowers looked alarmed, and I understood at once that she did not share my mother's Christian zeal.

"Well, that's a fine reason," Mrs. Flowers said, winking. Then to my mother: "Alice, I like Tom's haircut. Did you cut it?"

"Oh, no," my mother said. "Thank you, though. I take the boys to Olividatti's, down on McCorkle Avenue in Kanawha City." Then they began to talk in the foreign language of hair-styles and recipes and flower arrangements.

Why did I want to be in the Guinness Book of World Records? The question had never occurred to me. The only answer I could come up with was another question:

Didn't everybody?

WILD, WILD LIFE

Leonard railed at the television set. He jabbed at it with an invisible poker. Eyes tearing up, his voice trembling and exaggerated like an out-of-breath runner, he shouted, "I had a book, I don't know what it is, it's like Woodrow Wilson. Lieutenant commander! I can't find it, I can feel the heat right here."

Then in a flash he calmed down.

He or Enid kept the television on nearly twenty-four hours a day. They skipped through the channels, looking for anything offering a semblance of news. Fact after fact droned from the set: *Israel is the most successful nation in the world in increasing rainfall artificially. . . . One billion years ago the sun was twenty to thirty percent dimmer. . . . Donald Duck received two hundred ninety-one votes in the Swedish election for prime minister. . . . Hang gliders in Los Angeles are using their bird's-eye view to help local police and fire departments. . . .*

Sometimes lucidity swept over Leonard like a wave, and he looked at me to continue a conversation we'd never started:

"For fun we used to grease the trolley tracks on Meridian Street where it went uphill. It'd just spin its wheels. We'd stack carriages in front of a business. We put a cow in the church tower. I'll tell you, a horse-drawn carriage was better for dates. The horse knew the way home — you didn't have to pay attention to the driving."

Then Leonard's wild, frightening smile.

In the parking lot outside Pizza Hut John stepped on the heel of my shoe. My heel popped out. "Flat tire?" John asked.

I tried to slide back into my shoe without using my hands, which clapped and clapped.

"Knock, knock," John said.

"Who's there?" I answered.

My mother held the door to Pizza Hut open for us.

"Tom," he said.

"Forget it," I said. "Nothing doing."

CODEINE DIARY III

There is a sleep like the long dissolve
of bone into black earth. Each nurse carries
a paper cup, a syringe of that sleep . . .

But the chrysanthemums, and the trees outside
the window, say: You are never tired enough.

Your second breath says it, and the room's tick,
the star-tiled floor, the chalk walls
through the night hours. You lie listening

as though to a voice inside your voice, a lullaby
deep in the throat. Now a small snowfall.
Now a first blur of sun staining the window.

"I like it," Ellen said after hearing me read it aloud. "But
not every nurse carries sleep in her pocket like me. I'm the
keeper of sleep around here, buster."

About 10:00 P.M. I saw a commercial featuring a thin, large-breasted woman grinning suggestively at a man wearing a towel. The man was lathering himself with shaving cream. The woman seemed to like shaving cream a great deal. The very idea of shaving cream seemed exciting to her.

I thought about Laura Rhodes, who'd sent me a note during homeroom: "Diane thinks you're cute." I wanted to know if Laura thought I was cute. Diane was nice, but Laura was an eye-shadowed, earringed mystery; Laura wore a bra. If only Laura could see me lather myself with shaving cream . . .

I clapped and clapped. The commercial ran into Alan King's Wonderful World of Aggravation, "Part XII."

ARS MORIENDI

Death's presence is conspicuously muted in the hospital. You know that patients like yourself are dying around you, but you rarely see them, rarely encounter their death. The dying, like the dead, are elsewhere. When you do happen upon the death of another patient, it occurs at the expense of the hospital's carefully erected and maintained facade of relentless progress against the body's decay.

Late one night the elderly woman in the room next to mine died. I never saw her; I judged her age by her voice. Her voice was unmistakably the voice of an old woman, albeit loud and gravelly, a smoker's voice. Her voice carried into my room whenever she received visitors (usually a young woman I took to be her granddaughter) or spoke to the nurses.

Her doctors must have seen her death coming; late in the evening a minister was summoned to her room.

I heard the scrape of his chair as he dragged it toward her bed.

He introduced himself and said something I couldn't make out. Then he said, "Are you ready to be with the Lord your God? Are you ready, Mrs. ———?" He said her name — I'm sure it had three syllables — but I couldn't hear it.

"Oh yes," Mrs. Threesyllables said. "I'm saved."

The strength of her voice surprised me. Had her doctors been premature to summon the minister?

"Are you sure, Mrs. ———?" the minister asked. "If someone asked you how you knew you were saved, what would you tell that person?"

"I've been saved since I was a little girl."

"Would you say you were going to heaven?"

A pause. She seemed to search her mind for a forgotten theological distinction between being saved and going to heaven. "Yes, yes," she said.

"If that same someone asked you how you knew you were going to heaven, what would you say?"

"Because I'm a good person."

"Is it because God loves you?"

"Yes."

"And why does He love you?"

"Because I'm a good person." She sounded confused now, and impatient. Her voice was losing its strength.

The minister sighed. "What I need you to understand, Mrs. ———, is that we are all sinners in the sight of God. He loves us, yes. But He loves us even though we don't deserve His love. And before we can fully experience His love, we need to understand that we don't deserve Him, that we are saved by His grace alone. Do you understand that?"

"You're saying He doesn't love me?" the woman said angrily. "I know He loves me. He's loved me all my life."

"Yes, of course He does," the minister said, his voice quivering. "But I need you to understand that you don't deserve that love. It's His gift, through His Son, Jesus Christ. Have you acknowledged your sin and repented to His Son, Jesus Christ?"

"I was saved when I was a little girl."

"Yes, Mrs. ———, that's wonderful, but have you acknowledged your sin?"

"God loves me," she said sullenly. "God loves me. I'm a good person."

"Yes, of course you are. But— "

"Leave me alone. Go away."

Eventually he gave up and left her room, his footsteps shattering the hallway's quiet.

She died a few hours later.

Captain Kangaroo and Mr. Green Jeans blurred into Fred and Barney in the town of Bedrock, who blurred into Howard Sprague giving Goober an earful on Andy of Mayberry.

I clapped and clapped.

The phone rang three times and stopped.

"Can you get that?" John asked, smirking. He was watching TV with me.

"Very funny," I said.

"It's Grandma Roush," my mother yelled from the kitchen. "She wants to talk to Tom."

I let out an exaggerated sigh. Would no one take my world record attempt seriously? "Tell her I'm breaking a world record!" I yelled back.

It was a shocking response.

John's jaw dropped in disbelief.

"I WILL NOT TELL YOUR GRANDMOTHER THAT HER GRANDSON IS TOO BUSY TO TALK TO HER!" My mother stormed into the dialysis room. I looked at her sheepishly.

"Sorry," I said.

"Pick up that phone right now, young man. Got it? I don't care if you're running for president of the United States." She cooled down. As a compromise, she said, "John can hold the phone to your ear."

"Okay," I said as she left the room.

John's face twisted into a parody of excessive politeness. "That's right," he said. "John can hold the phone to your ear."

Warily, I let John hold the phone to my ear.

"Hello, Grandma?" I said.

"Now, Tom," said my grandmother, "what in the dickens are you doing?"

My clapping almost drowned out her voice, so I nearly shouted into the phone: "I'm trying to break a record for the Guinness Book of World Records!"

"The what?"

"It's a book with all the records of the world in it. Like the tallest man, the biggest kidney stone. All kinds of stuff. I'm going to clap my hands longer than fourteen hours and six minutes."

John started poking me in the ribs with his free hand. He whispered, "Biggest kidney stone! What a dork." I jerked away but kept clapping. John held up his hands as if in surrender. "Truce," he said, holding the phone to my ear again.

Glaring at John, I said, "What was that, Grandma?"

"Your mother tells me you're not doing so well in school. Is it because you're thinking too much about this stunt of yours?"

"I can do better in school." I said it to placate her, knowing that six words was all it would take.

John rolled his eyes.

"All right, then," my grandmother said. "You do that. Let me talk to your mother now, honey."

John hung up the phone. "Bet you five dollars she called you 'honey,'" he said.

FUZZY LOGIC

Some people will do anything for attention," Balazs said, leading Bill and Caryn into my room at the hospital. Balazs was an editor at *Mathematical Reviews*. He edited the sections on functional analysis and operator theory. He and two Fuzzy Sets, Bill and Caryn, had come to see how I was doing. Their visit was well timed. I was feeling good, humming along on codeine, ready to catch up on the shenanigans at *MR*.

"Look who's here," I said. "Boy, it's great to see you guys."

Caryn smiled and walked over to the window. Bill, inspecting my right leg, said, "I guess the crazed bleeder jock was at it again."

"Just call me Air Gimp," I said. "I'm working on a deal with Nike."

"Cool," Caryn said. "You can see the river. Terry and Nancy wanted to come, but they had a supervisors' meeting. This is from Terry."

Caryn handed me a sheet of computer paper. I held it to my ear, shaking it gently like a wrapped present to guess its contents.

"Just read it," Caryn said.

It was Terry's current finger.plan. It poked glorious fun at *Hymning the Kanawha,* my first book of poems. The book had come out during my last episode with a broken ankle. That fact, combined with the inherently quixotic nature of

publishing a book of poems with a small press, presented her
with plenty of comic buttons to push:

```
                    ACT NOW!
        GET YOUR VERY OWN, MADE IN USA,
  OFFICIAL "Hymning the Kanawha" TOUR JACKET!!

  Featuring
  —Salmon lettering on teal
  —Over left breast:

              HYMNING THE KANAWHA
                   Tour '89
  —Across back yoke: "a careful, human voice"
  —Italian styling, Velcro'd shoulder pads
  —Lining embroidered with official Tom An-
    drews autograph in repeated pattern
  —Children's sizes XS-S-M-L, adult sizes
    VP-P-S-M-L-XL-XXL

  Send $139.95 to
          TSHco Diversitronics
          701 N. Fourth Ave., Dept. TCA
          Ann Arbor, MI 48104
```

"I want one!" I hooted. "Does the author get a discount?
Maybe I'll get one for my grandmother, too."

"I bet you can work something out with Terry," Caryn said.

I noticed the pin Caryn was wearing on her black turtle-
neck sweater. It was one of Terry's. She made pins modeled after Max Ernst collages and Joseph Cornell boxes and sold
them at a store on Main Street. This one featured a tiny green
wooden car pasted onto a background of Beijing's imperial

palace. The silhouette of a dancing woman loomed over the palace and the car. "Great pin," I said.

"Hey, thanks," Caryn said.

"So," Bill said. "I bet you're dying to know all the *MR* gossip." Bill had a face like a basset hound's: immeasurably sad and eliciting. You wanted to do whatever he said.

"I am, I am," I said.

"The big news," Bill said, "is that Anne-Marie balled out Walter for being rude to the copyeditors."

"Really?" I said.

"Yeah," Bill said. "Apparently she really let him have it. Barbara said she wanted to crawl under the table."

Caryn said, "I have trouble with Anne-Marie, but she does wear a Swatch. She can't be all bad."

Balazs said, "What is it with you and these Swatch watches?"

"Let me tell you," Caryn said. She exaggerated, knowingly, her own passionate interest and knowledge. "The Swatch, to quote the nineteen eighty-eight Swatch Museum catalog, has become a symbol of youth, of individualism, of uncomplicated joie de vivre. Its success is due to — feel free to stop me at any point."

Balazs said, "Do they pay you a salary or do you work on commission?"

"That's a secret," Caryn said. "Can I interest you in a Gray Memphis?" She pulled up her left sleeve, exposing a Swatch watch with a gray plastic band and with green and red hands. The watch's face was a cut-up series of geometric forms and faux surfaces in black and white. "Nineteen eighty-four," Caryn said. "The second year Swatches were available in the U.S."

"That's a nice one," I said.

"Or" — Caryn raised her chin coquettishly and extended her right arm, limp-wristed, toward Bill — "maybe you prefer the Transparent Jelly Fish? Oops." She had forgotten to pull up her right sleeve, which she now did, exposing another Swatch. This one was made entirely of clear plastic except for the hands, which were red, blue, and yellow. One could see the inner mechanism, the tiny cogs notching on and on, the tiny coil and copper plates, the tiny battery.

"Looks like one of those transparent telephones," Balazs said.

Bill said, "It'd make me nervous to have so much of my watch out in the open like that. Has it no shame? Besides, it demystifies itself. There are some mysteries I want to preserve."

"From the man who still wears bell-bottoms," Caryn said. "It's okay with us, you know, if you want to wear your leisure suits, too."

"Even my lime green one?" Bill said.

"Especially the lime green one," Caryn said. "That way, when you spill Jell-O on it, you won't have to do anything."

Somehow the conversation segued to a little boy who lived next door to Bill. The boy had two invisible friends. "Their names are Fool and Ash," Bill said. "*Fool* I could understand. But *Ash!* I asked him where *Ash* came from and he said, 'From the fire.' 'What fire,' I said. And he goes, 'From the fire at the bottom of everything.'"

"Come on," I said. "You're making this up."

"I'm serious," Bill said. "I couldn't believe it, either. I asked the kid's parents if they'd been reading Heracleitus aloud or something. The father said no, but the mother said, "Well, you know how Heracleitus is in the air these days.'"

"Come on," I said.

"I'm serious," Bill said.

"Come on," I said.

Balazs pulled his wallet out of his back pocket and searched through it. "I almost forgot to give this to you," he said, finding a folded-up piece of paper and handing it to me.

"I thought you would like this. I found it in a biography of Stan Ulam."

It was a Xerox of a photograph of a memorandum Ulam had written with another mathematician, J. Carson Mark, while the two were working at Los Alamos.

December 18, 1947

A & S Memorandum No. 10742
To All Concerned:

For your convenience and ready reference, we have had prepared the following list of the numbers 0–100 (inclusive) in alphabetical order.

12, 8, 18, 80, 88, 85, 84, 89, 81, 87, 86, 83, 82, 11, 15, 50, 58, 55, 54, 59, 51, 57, 56, 53, 52, 5, 40, 48, 45, 44, 49, 41, 47, 46, 43, 42, 4, 14, 9, 19, 90, 98, 95, 94, 99, 91, 97, 96, 93, 92, 1, 100, 7, 17, 70, 78, 75, 74, 79, 71, 77, 76, 73, 72, 6, 16, 60, 68, 65, 64, 69, 61, 67, 66, 63, 62, 13, 30, 38, 35, 34, 39, 31, 37, 36, 33, 32, 3, 12, 20, 28, 25, 24, 29, 21, 27, 26, 23, 22, 2, 0.

For the Associate Director

"This is great," I said, staring at the memo. "I love catalogs and minutiae like this."

Caryn said, "When I showed it to Walter, he said it was the best thing that ever came out of Los Alamos."

"Something's not right, though," I said. "Right?"

"Aha!" Balazs said to Bill and Caryn. "Let's see if he catches it."

"Is it just me or should it start with eight?" I said.

"The first twelve is meant to be read as *a dozen*," Balazs said.

"Oh, I see," I said. "There are two *twelves*."

"And . . . ," Balazs said.

"And? And what?" I said.

"There's no *ten*," Caryn said.

"Mister Copyeditor loses the prize," Balazs said. "Your punishment is keeping your job."

Bill said, "Speaking of which, I have to get back to the office."

"Me, too," Caryn said. "It looks like you're doing okay?"

"I'm doing okay," I said. "Thanks a lot for dropping by. I really appreciate it."

"Anytime," Bill said. "Well, no, not *any* time. Some times are never good for me. Two in the morning, for instance. Of course, I hope for your sake there won't be another time. That would be — "

"Let's go, Bill," Caryn said, grabbing Bill by the arm and leading him out of the room. "See you later."

Balazs said he could stay a little while longer. I was pleased. Balazs was the friendliest *MR* editor. He came to *MR* from Romania, where he grew up and went to school. One of his peers in his Ph.D. program in mathematics had been the daughter of Nicolae Ceauşescu, Romania's brutal dictator. Balazs told me stories of being in a car several times with Ceauşescu and the daughter. On one ride they passed the construction site of what was to be a ten-story building. The foundation had been laid and the first four floors constructed. Balazs remembered Ceauşescu's having the chauffeur stop the car and barking out the window to the foreman, "No more floors! That's high enough!" Other times he would yell, "Tear it down, it's ugly!" After years of such drive-by second-guessings and demolitions, Balazs said, Bucharest began to look like a toy city into which some kid had tossed firecrackers.

"I'm writing a story," Balazs said after Bill and Caryn left the room.

"Tell me about it," I said.

Balazs's story was about a software salesman in Bucharest. The salesman's fiancée of several years leaves him on a Saturday night. The salesman is devastated, but the thing is, he has a career-making meeting on Monday morning with a government official. By Monday he needs to be over his grief. On his cracked apartment wall he draws up a schedule so that he can work through the five stages of grief in thirty hours, or six hours per stage.

"That's all I've got so far," Balazs said.

"I love it," I said. "Absolutely. I can't wait to read it."

"I've got lots of ideas. My problem is, I don't know how to flesh out the events. Stories come easily, but the writing — that's another matter. I've been reading *At the Bottom of the River,* by Jamaica Kincaid. Everything flows so smoothly. You never see her working. In the best of all possible worlds, that's how I'd like to write."

"Wow. I didn't know you were so serious about writing," I said. I'd meant it as a compliment, but Balazs felt attacked.

"Why? Because I'm a mathematician? You think C. P. Snow was right about the two cultures? You're a mathematician; you write."

"I'm not a mathematician and I'm hardly a writer. But what I meant was — "

"I find that scientists keep up with the humanities much more than humanities professors keep up with scientific work."

"I'm sorry, Balazs. I didn't mean to offend you. What I meant was, I'm surprised you're so serious about writing *not* because you're a mathematician but because it takes so much time and energy, and I know how busy you are."

"That's true," Balazs said, calming down. "That's true. That's why I'll never be good at it."

"What do you mean?" I said. "That's going to be a great story."

"Think of it this way. What if you decided you wanted to start publishing in the *Journal of Operator Theory*. How much time would it take you to get there?"

"Good point, Balazs. Good point."

AFFIDAVIT

STATE OF WEST VIRGINIA
COUNTY OF KANAWHA, TO WIT:

THOMAS C. ANDREWS of 1714 Rolling Hills Circle,
Charleston, Kanawha County, West Virginia 25314, being
first duly sworn upon his oath, deposes and says that he is
eleven (11) years of age; that his birthday is April 30, 1961;
that he is God-fearing and sensible to the meaning and
seriousness of making this statement under oath even
though a minor; that on the 15th day of November, 1972,
he undertook to and did establish a new world's record for
continuous hand-clapping; that in the Guinness Book of
World Records, *Revised American Edition, compiled by*
Norris and Ross McWhirter, *copyrighted 1972 by Sterling*
Publishing Co., Inc., of 419 Park Avenue South, New York,
New York 10016, at pages 425–427, the record for
continuous hand-clapping is set forth as being fourteen (14)
hours and six (6) minutes; that on the 15th day of
November, 1972, he commenced clapping his hands at
precisely eight (8:00) o'clock, a.m., eastern standard time, as
shown by a General Electric eight-inch (8") commercial-
style electric clock; that he continued clapping his hands at a
varying rate which averaged one hundred and twenty (120)
claps per minute throughout the day, the minimum rate
being approximately one hundred (100) claps per minute;
that said hand-clapping was done in the residence of his
parents in which he resided, the audibility level being
sufficient to be heard therein; that he ceased clapping his
hands at ten thirty-one (10:31) o'clock, p.m., eastern
standard time, on said 15th day of November, 1972, as

shown by said General Electric clock, which said clock remained running throughout the period of time of the hand-clapping herein described; that the total elapsed time of said continuous hand-clapping conducted by him was fourteen (14) hours and thirty-one (31) minutes, being twenty-five (25) minutes longer than the previous world record as shown on pages 425–427 of said Guinness Book of World Records; *that throughout said period of fourteen (14) hours and thirty-one (31) minutes he was observed and in the presence of one or more of the following persons: his mother, Alice R. Andrews, of 1714 Rolling Hills Circle, Charleston, Kanawha County, West Virginia 25314; his father, H. Raymond Andrews, Jr., of 1714 Rolling Hills Circle, Charleston, Kanawha County, West Virginia 25314; his brother, John H. Andrews, of 1714 Rolling Hills Circle, Charleston, Kanawha County, West Virginia 25314, who is sixteen (16) years of age; Mrs. Mary Colbert, of 5312 Alden Street, South Charleston, Kanawha County, West Virginia 25303; Leonard Sargeant III, of 1726 Rolling Hills Circle, Charleston, Kanawha County, West Virginia 25314; and Mrs. Eleanor Flowers, of 1982 Parkwood Road, Charleston, Kanawha County, West Virginia 25314; that at least one of said persons listed was always present and observing him throughout said period; and that no period of time occurred during said fourteen (14) hours and thirty-one (31) minutes when he was not in the presence of and observed by at least one of said persons listed; and that said hand-clapping continued unabated during and throughout the said fourteen (14) hours and thirty-one (31) minutes.*

Dated this 17th day of November, 1972.

THOMAS C. ANDREWS

Taken, sworn to, and acknowledged before me, a Notary Public in and for the county and state aforesaid, this 17th day of November, 1972.

Given under my hand and notarial seal this 17th day of November, 1972.

My commission expires January 21, 1974.

MAE U. ADAMS
Notary Public, Kanawha County,
West Virginia

CODEINE DIARY IV

At any time of the day or night, somewhere in the hospital, Muzak is playing. Right now I hear a neurasthenic version of "Every Breath You Take" by the Police. It makes me think of a line from Confessions of an English Opium Eater: "The tyranny of the violin."

The thing is, intense pain demands that you doubt whether it exists, whether you exist. Are you making it all up, a bizarre self-flagellar hallucination? And the world: does this brown table exist? (Is this brown table brown?) That orange vinyl chair? The star-tiled floor? Does the pain come from them, or from me?

Pain seizes you but you can't say it inhabits your body. Pain is not in your body, and neither are you. You are not in your body, neither are you anywhere else. Pain displaces you. Yes. But there's no content to pain. It offers nothing, not even itself. It's a vacancy, a namelessness your body plunges into, and meanwhile, where are you?

This morning I missed the plastic urinal, fouling the sheets.

———

Not unto judgment nor unto condemnation be my partaking of thy Holy Mysteries, O Lord, but unto the healing of the soul and body.

———

Outside, snow's falling again. The loyal and fragmented snow. Bright looming dark.

———

"For instance, I don't know how to sweep," says Phil Donahue.
"I'll teach you," says the guest sociologist.

———

This bed as embryonic world. Its vast cerulean distances, its equatorial thickets. Regions of hissing ash, monsoons, midnight suns. To move my leg a few inches: an emigration from Tashkent to Bogotá. To turn over: an impossible odyssey, a tale for Jules Verne.

———

The narcosis of television. Watching TV for hours is like taking a great deal of codeine when you have no pain. The more you take it, the more you develop a need for it that can never be satisfied. Like pain, watching TV for hours has no content. Unlike pain, it kills time. Which, as Ezra Pound said, is fine, if you like your time dead.

———

Carrieless hours.

———

The sound of a dog barking ferociously.

———

John, you're vague as mist, dressed up in dew, smoke. I keep seeing you, haunting the hawthorn trees within earshot of the riverbank. Asking nothing.

Dear Tom,

It was certainly nice to read that you have broken the world's record in clapping. Keep your Dad busy getting that affidavit recorded.

We used to enjoy seeing how your Dad recorded you in your annual picture for Christmas. The last few years we had lost touch.

Congratulations again. Everyone is very proud of you.

> *Sincerely,*
> *The Ripley Fishers*

THE ISLAND OF DR. H

She came and went, my hematologist, her schedule as inscrutable as turbulence. Sometimes half a dozen interns clustered around her. They looked like children, rich white kids playing doctor, stethoscopes dangling absurdly from their gleaming necks.

The thought of my hematologist's (whom I'll call Dr. H) visiting me brought mixed comfort. In the past I'd been treated by a few doctors whose ruling dictum for administering care to patients was a variation on the Victorian method of parenthood: patients should be seen and not heard. Dr. H, thank God, was not one of them. She wanted to see and hear patients. But she wanted to see and hear them, it seemed, as long as they assented to her first thoughts about their condition. She confidently applied Allen Ginsberg's often-repeated statement on the creative process, "First thought, best thought," to hematology. The results were frightening, at least to me. Each question I asked appeared to first irritate and then anger her, which in turn irritated and angered me and made me want to ask more questions. It was hardly a fair fight. When I had persisted in questioning her (in my opinion) recklessly casual optimism about HIV and factor VIII, I thought she was going to give me a bleed herself. I provoked her anger — or something approaching anger, anger watered down with displeasure. Her subsequent visits meant tap-dancing around our mutual volatility while at the same time asserting my need to take responsibility for my healing.

I knew, of course, that her anger had nothing to do with me personally. Carrie helped remind me of that after each appointment or checkup. *Impersonal hostility* was a catchall phrase Carrie used when a waiter was rude to her, when someone stole a parking space from her, when a librarian looked down his or her nose at her. "Impersonal hostility," Carrie had said when she spoke with Dr. H on the phone or in person. "Highly paid, highly rewarded impersonal hostility."

As a patient I want to take responsibility for my healing, working in cooperation with a doctor. We are to be co-conspirators in this raid on illness. Or, to use a less aggressive metaphor, we'll be part of a cleanup crew assigned to the vagrant blood spilled in my body. Physicians who cannot accept this relationship offer the patient a no-win proposition. The patient can agree to do whatever the physician says without question, thereby abandoning his or her instinctive intelligence, curiosity, and passion. Or the patient can "fight" the physician's imperial posture, demanding to be an equal partner, knowing that doing so may raise the physician's ire. In the first option, the patient must live with bad faith, its humiliating self-alienation: *acting dumb*. In the second, which is preferable and which demands considerable courage, the patient must trust the physician to provide effective care even while expressing hostility to the patient. Such trust, however, may not exist.

I trusted my hematologist. But I wanted evidence that she paused to consider, scrutinize, bring the weight of her experience upon, revise when necessary — reenvision from different angles — her thoughts to arrive at my prognosis. I wanted evidence that she'd seen *me*, and not simply my chart. I wanted more time, but not *much* more time, a few minutes at most. As Anatole Broyard wrote in *Intoxicated by My Illness*:

I see no reason for my doctor to love me — nor would I expect him to suffer with me. I wouldn't demand a lot of my doctor's time: I just wish he would brood on my situation for perhaps five minutes, that he would give me his whole mind just once, be bonded with me for a brief space, survey my soul as well as my flesh, to get at my illness, for each man is ill in his own way.

I would love a hematologist to survey my soul as well as my flesh to get at my illness, but I'll settle for the extra five minutes.

I wouldn't demand a lot of my doctor's time . . . perhaps five minutes. Personal narratives of illness repeat this complaint so often as to be a prerequisite to the genre. In *A Whole New Life,* Reynolds Price describes the moment when two doctors gave him the news that a snakelike tumor had likely taken up residence inside his spinal cord. Price was in a stretcher in the hallway of Duke University Hospital. "What would those two splendidly trained men have lost," Price wonders, "if they'd waited to play their trump till I was back in the private room . . . ?"

It might have taken the doctors five minutes longer; and minutes are scarce, I know, in their crowded days. I also know that for doctors who work, from dawn to night, in the same drab halls, it all no doubt feels like one room. But any patient can tell them it's not. . . .

I could, of course, have chosen to see a different hematologist. But hemophilia is not a glamour disease. It doesn't attract stars, the most ambitious and brilliant medical students. Dr. H was one of the few stars of hematology. She was the expert. She was the hematologist to whom other hematologists deferred. The prospect of fighting with her and possibly raising her ire notwithstanding, I wanted her expertise. Besides, I still had hope of educating *her*, of doctoring her in the most heathful way of treating me and other hemophiliacs. Convalescence is a two-way street. I wanted to be an ambitious patient.

8:00 A.M. *The first awkward tentative claps.*

"So you're really going through with this," John said.

We were in the dialysis room, the room with the television. Captain Kangaroo strolled with Mr. Green Jeans through the Treasure House. Grandfather Clock eyed them wisely, impartially.

"I can't believe you still watch that crap," John said.

It took me a second to realize I didn't have to stop clapping to talk. "Do you mind?" I said. "I'm breaking a world record here."

KON-TIKI, PAGE 107

The next night was still worse; the seas grew higher instead of going down. Two hours on end of struggling with the steering oar was too long; a man was not much use in the second half of his watch, and the seas got the better of us and hurled us round and sideways, while the water poured on board. Then we changed over to one hour at the helm and an hour and a half's rest. So the first sixty hours passed, in one continuous struggle against a chaos of waves that rushed upon us, one after another, without cessation. High waves and low waves, pointed waves and round waves, slanting waves and waves on top of other waves.

Dear Tom,

*Try to come out if you can, but if you can't that's o.k. I
can play till about 4:00 or 5:00. I hope you come out.
Will you walk with me today? Circle   YES   NO*

*I think you are the nicest boy over in Rolling Hills. I'm
going to try to get you something.*

Love, Diane

*P.S. Write back if you want to. Don't let anybody else see
this, except Nan if you want to. Or Laura. I just showed
Nan and Laura. Do you mind? Circle   YES   NO*

Answer questions and give back, please.

ONE HUNDRED SPECTACULAR
SOUND EFFECTS

From a hemophiliac's point of view, the story of hemophilia is, in the end, a story about pain: how to withstand it, how to outguess it, how to distract yourself from it, how to embrace it.

Pain twisted me literally and mentally. Two days into the bleed my right knee became locked at a forty-five-degree angle. Blood rushed the joints' interiors, filled them, and kept rushing. Once a joint was full, there was nowhere for oncoming blood to go; it simply pressed and pressed against the nerve endings. Soon, I knew, the muscles in my leg would atrophy to the shape of the bent leg.

"Straighten your leg as far as you comfortably can," my hematologist said during one of her visits. "But don't push it. What we want to avoid is another bleed inside the joints."

Yes.

Yes.

—————

Pain was acutest during the last half hour of a dose of codeine. I was lucky to have Carrie to help me make the transition from one dose to another. Carrie was with me, often, during the day. We held hands. Hours passed. Inevitably one of us gripped tighter than the other. Usually it was me. Without thinking, I'd squeeze her long thin hand until her fingers were scrunched together, pinky ducked under the ring finger, like asparagus stalks bound by a rubber band. When I realized what I was doing, I weakened my grip. Carrie interpreted this as a desire to remove my hand, and took her hand away.

"No," I said, adding my superfluous voice.

———

Carrie often read aloud to me, urging my mind to drift on her voice like a kite on a string. When I was lucky, and could concentrate on Carrie's voice, she kept me hovering far enough away to find relief and yet close enough to hear her utter a small handful of the world's intelligible contours. She read poets: Jean Valentine, Wallace Stevens, Benjamin Péret. She read books crowded with physical details, like *Kon-Tiki* or an old high school science textbook called *The Physical Universe*. Sometimes she simply read aloud the contents of a cassette she'd found called *100 Spectacular Sound Effects*.

"Eleven. Swarm of bees," Carrie said.

Pause.

"Twelve. One cricket."

Pause.

"Thirteen. Bullfrog."

Pause.

"Fourteen. Single bee."

Pause.

"Fifteen. Windshield wipers."

Pause.

"Sixteen. Mantel clock."

Pause.

"Seventeen. Slot maching, coins falling."

Pause.

"Eighteen. Heavy traffic."

If Carrie read this to me when I was well into a dose of codeine, the only thing tethering me to the hospital bed was my IV line.

––––––––

Sometimes, when we were both feeling up to it, Carrie and I would read plays together. Samuel Beckett's *Waiting for Godot* was nearly always at the top of our list. One of the transformative reading experiences of my life was looking up *Waiting for Godot* at the Kanawha County Public Library in Charleston when I was eighteen. I'm not sure what made me want to look it up. Probably I'd run across a reference to it in an essay by S. J. Perelman — the source of many treasures in those days. When I found the play in the stacks, I was thrilled by how short it was. Literature with a capital *L* evoked images of interminably long, deathly boring works. (Later, in college, reading John Berryman's fourteenth "Dream Song" brought a shiver of pleasure: "Literature bores me, especially great literature.")

Opening the play was like taking cotton out of my ears. I couldn't believe what I was hearing. Beckett's lines were somehow utterly beautiful *and* funny, a combination I'd never encountered before in any art. His timing was as good as Laurel and Hardy's. His phrases and cadences were bewitched by a mathematical precision. If this was literature, I remember thinking, I was hooked. Moreover, if *Waiting for Godot* was literature, then maybe even "Laurel and Hardy: An Oral Hystery" could be affirmed within the generous shadow it cast.

Carrie and I often began with a favorite moment in the play, an exchange in the second act when Vladimir and Estragon's music-hall banter soars with lyricism:

ESTRAGON: In the meantime let us try and converse
   calmly, since we are incapable of keeping silent.
VLADIMIR: You're right, we're inexhaustible.
ESTRAGON: It's so we won't think.
VLADIMIR: We have that excuse.
ESTRAGON: It's so we won't hear.
VLADIMIR: We have our reasons.
ESTRAGON: All the dead voices.
VLADIMIR: They make a sound like wings.
ESTRAGON: Like leaves.
VLADIMIR: Like sand.
ESTRAGON: Like leaves.

   Silence.

VLADIMIR: They all speak at once.
ESTRAGON: Each one to itself.

   Silence.

VLADIMIR: Rather they whisper.
ESTRAGON: They rustle.
VLADIMIR: They murmur.
ESTRAGON: They rustle.

   Silence.

Waiting for Godot had become part of our regular hospital survivor kit, so to speak. An actor once asked Beckett the meaning of the play. "Oh," Beckett said, "it's just me and my wife." (A reference perhaps to the harrowing days when Beckett and his wife, as members of the Resistance in occupied France, were forced to flee to the south of the country on foot.) In the hospital, it had become me and my wife, too.

CARRIE: What do they say?
TOM: They talk about their lives.
CARRIE: To have lived is not enough.
TOM: They have to talk about it.
CARRIE: To be dead is not enough for them.
TOM: It is not sufficient.

Silence.

CARRIE: They make a noise like feathers.
TOM: Like leaves.
CARRIE: Like ashes.
TOM: Like leaves.

Long silence.

"John," I said, still clapping at 3:55 P.M., nearly eight hours into the record, "who's George McGovern?"

It was a risky question. It proved I knew nothing. Sometimes John allowed me to know nothing without punishing me, sometimes he'd answer a question like the one I'd just asked, but I shouldn't have tested him, not now, when my clapping was like a personal assault on his ears.

I asked the question softly, so he'd hear it only if he was listening hard. As soon as I'd said it, though, I knew I'd made a mistake. After eight hours, this clapping business, as my mother affectionately called it, lulled me into lowering my defenses in the ongoing war of wits with John. One slip like this could shift the balance of power miserably. My face reddened.

I clapped louder, and waited.

John hadn't heard my question.

THE LOST FISHING NOTEBOOKS OF
SRINIVASA RAMANUJAN

When I was in the waiting room, I had tried to dredge up a theorem to distract me from pain. I loved working on difficult mathematical problems. I loved the way my mind *felt*—intensely focused, alert, transfixed—as I worked. It was very much like working on a poem, but without the sometimes maddening, sometimes delighting, always politically and emotionally charged imprecision of words. No wonder Paul Valéry longed for his poems to embody "the solidity of certain pages of algebra."

Working on a problem, you feel the answer moving in you, an obscure presence in your body. It starts in the back of the knees, then rises slowly into the spine, traversing blood and muscle tissue. The answer is patient, shy, fragile. If coaxed too soon up the spinal column into the brain, it dissolves like a sugar cube in hot tea. This all takes place, mind you, while you are beating your head against the wall. You feel the answer nestling there in the knees, in the spine. The excitement is tremendous as the solution inches upward, intact, into your consciousness. That's when it is easiest to lose concentration, to make a mistake. You anticipate the joy of solving the problem rather than keep working on it. But when you do solve it, it is as though your body, which moments before was a hugely complicated knot, is untied quickly with a single firm tug. Then—to shift from a sexual to an electrical metaphor—your body seems to buzz a little, to tap into a low galvanic current.

For me, mathematics means entrance into unseen worlds composed of such exquisite beauty, radiant structure, and interpenetrating detail that I am nearly breathless when I am ushered into them. Mathematics also means an impossible freedom from circumstance — from bleeds, from habits of mind, from various mundane struggles, from limitations of every stripe. But I am never able to focus on a mathematical problem during bleeds. I am never able to experience that alertness, that transfixion.

But this day I wanted to change that. Could I bring the quality of attention required to work through a theorem while my leg swelled and hissed at me and I waited for my next dose of codeine?

My work at *MR* put me in daily contact with gifted mathematicians around the world. Despite — or perhaps because of — the fact that they moved through the material world as through dense fog, unsure of their footing, unable to pause for more than a few minutes from whatever problem was currently obsessing them, the mathematicians I met and corresponded with were seeking something beyond themselves, something unprecedented. In that sense I saw them as heroic.

Now I wanted to breathe on the heroic.

I recalled a theorem of Srinivasa Ramanujan's, the great Indian mathematician. It worked its magic, filling me, as it always did, with awe and with something like sublimity:

$$(1.11) \, \frac{1}{1+} \, \frac{e^{-2\pi}}{1+} \, \frac{e^{-4\pi}}{1+} = \left\{ \sqrt{\left(\frac{5+\sqrt{5}}{2}\right)} - \frac{\sqrt{5}+1}{2} \right\} e^{2/5\pi}$$

I kept this theorem taped to the wall in front of my desk at work, flanked by a haunting poem of Jean Valentine's called "After Elegies" and a black-and-white photo of Carrie smoking. The theorem fascinated and troubled me. Sometimes looking at it filled me with a strange calm. Other times it induced vertigo. Sometimes it was like music — slow, grave music that occasionally and without warning erupted into passionate, dissonant bursts, crisp glissandos and arpeggios: a Bach partita metamorphosed into a Schoenberg gigue. Sometimes the theorem, like music, entered me and spread inside me, enlarging my sense of what is possible; enlarging *me*. More often than not, though, it remained as mute as the wall it was taped to.

I stared at the theorem every day at work. I tried not to let my colleagues catch me gawking. Like Robert Benchley hiding his volumes of Proust and Joyce from his *New Yorker* colleagues (who let him know he was supposed to urbanely savage the pretentions of such writers, not admire them), I stared at the theorem furtively, with fear and trembling, as though it were an entry in a censored devotional. Looking at it, watching the gull-flight of Ramanujan's intuition on the page, satisfied some itch or hunger that could not be satisfied in any other way.

That I could remember the theorem as I lay there in my bed in the hospital surprised and encouraged me. Did this mean I was learning to "conquer" pain somehow, distract myself from it sufficiently to give my mind a measure of independence?

As soon as I remembered the theorem, I forgot it entirely. It slipped from my consciousness without a trace. I couldn't lift it back to memory no matter how strenuously I tried. Into its place hurried another theorem that I also stared at every day, though this one I kept in my top desk drawer, on top of a pile of manila envelopes, so that all I had to do was pull open the drawer and look down at the efficient viper's nest of symbols and numbers that made up the following differential equation:

$$\frac{d(N_{14}I_{14})}{d+} = (1 - p)b \frac{\Sigma N_i(I_i + A_{i1} + \cdots + A_{i\ell})}{\Sigma N_i}$$

$$\frac{d(N_{14}A_{14,1})}{d+} = \frac{\Sigma N_i(I_i + A_{i1} + \cdots + A_{i\ell})}{\Sigma N_i} - \gamma_{14}N_{14}A_{14,1}$$

$$\vdots$$

$$\frac{d(N_{14}A_{14,m})}{d+} = \gamma_{14,m-1}N_{14}A_{14,m-1} - \gamma_{14,m}N_{14}A_{14,m}$$

This equation was from a paper on the transmission dynamics of HIV. It modeled the probability of infected blood from a given group of people (here denoted by i) within a given population. (The probability is I_iN_i/N, where N is the population size.)

Hidden somewhere within that equation was a symbol representing me — a symbol representing hemophiliacs who received repeated infusions between 1978 and 1985 and yet miraculously, bewilderingly, were HIV-negative.

I could not find that symbol no matter how long I stared.

Philadelphia Enquirer   November 28, 1972

MARTIN BORMANN REPORTED ALIVE IN SOUTH AMERICA
CHAMPION'S ROUTES TO GLORY

And sometimes champions have highly developed imagina-tions that help them in their quest for glory. Tom Andrews, only 11, of Charleston, W.Va., applauded without interrup-tion for 14 hours 31 minutes. His father, Ray, so attested in an affidavit he sent to The Guinness Book of World Records.

VACANCY IN THE PARK
BY WALLACE STEVENS

March . . . Someone has walked across the snow,
Someone looking for he knows not what.

It is like a boat that has pulled away
From a shore at night and disappeared.

It is like a guitar left on a table
By a woman, who has forgotten it.

It is like the feeling of a man
Come back to see a certain house.

The four winds blow through the rustic arbor,
Under its mattresses of vines.

Read that one again," I said. "Do you mind?"
Seventy-four words in a certain order, as miraculous as
the whirligig beetle.

"Sure. No problem," Carrie said.

John and I were in the driveway waiting for my mother to take us to Pizza Hut.

I snorted and hawked and spat onto the driveway, still clapping. Sometimes I could fire a trembling projectile of spit as casually as Willie Stargell. But this time the spit didn't leave my mouth cleanly; it dribbled down my lower lip and chin. I tried to suck it back up into my mouth. No good. I tried wiping my chin in between claps. Then I got spit on my hands and tried to wipe them, between claps, on my pants leg.

John was cracking up, laughing and bending double. When my mother walked out of the house, she saw me trying to wipe spit on John's back while I was still clapping and John was dodging me a like a toreador.

CODEINE DIARY V

Today an ice storm! What I wouldn't give to walk out into the glittering field below my window. Each blade of grass, I imagine, is encased in a tiny vial of ice. Each twig and stem. Even a pile of dogshit is a glittering wonder. The branches of the elm and maple trees bend and creak with the sudden weight of ice. A few are bent so far that when the wind blows they sweep the ground, clattering icy brooms. Others snap and fall with sounds like explosions. I imagine stamping across a lawn or field in snow boots, jumping up and down, the frozen grass and leaves breaking and cracking under my feet like fine china.

Jesus said: Split a stick. I will be inside.

Reading Kon-Tiki. The hospital sways and creaks like a ship at sea, cresting a wave before plunging down the other side, cresting, plunging. Creaking. The floor tilts one way, then another. As in old cartoons, nurses and orderlies wear suction cups on the soles of their shoes to keep their balance. Doctors hover, imperceptibly, half an inch above the floor. Here comes a technician pushing a cart of X rays and blood samples. He takes his hands off the cart, and the cart accelerates from him as the hospital crashes down a wave. The technician stares at the cart, his mouth a wide hole. Another wave.

The cart rushes back toward the technician, pursuing him, picking up speed. He runs, or tries to run, away from the cart, his speed hampered pathetically by the suction cups on his shoes. His mouth a wide hole . . .

―――――

The riffled sea of my sheets.

―――――

Wash what is soiled, water what is dry, heal what is wounded, bend what is rigid, warm what is cold, find what is lost.

―――――

The world is a flushed, iridescent leg.

Charleston Daily Mail   Wednesday November 22, 1972

OAKWOOD PUPIL BREAKS WORLD CLAPPING
RECORD — EARNS APPLAUSE

*Oakwood Elementary celebrated two Toms today —
Thanksgiving's Tom Turkey and record-breaker Tom Andrews, a fifth grader.*

*Andrews, 11-year-old son of Mr. and Mrs. H. Raymond
Andrews of 1714 Rolling Hills Circle, spent Nov. 15 hand
clapping for 14¹/₂ hours, breaking a previous world record.
He was out of school for a parent–teacher conference day.*

According to the Guinness Book of World Records, *two Brit-
ish teenagers in 1968 clapped 25 minutes less than Andrews.*

*"Tom went to school today on a cloud," his mother com-
mented about her son's recent publicity. He received classmates'
recognition during a Thanksgiving assemby this afternoon.*

*Mrs. Andrews explained that the youngster has been fasci-
nated with the* Guinness book, *which he received for his 10th
birthday, and decided two records he could beat were omelet
making and clapping. She encouraged the latter.*

*"I knew all along he could break the record. He's a very
persistent child," Mrs. Andrews reported. She said she helped
him eat pizza and drink soup and milkshakes through a straw
during his daylong ordeal. His father, an attorney for the Co-
lumbia Gas Co. of West Virginia, prepared a detailed affidavit
for submission to Guinness publishers.*

"*The book doesn't tell you what to do to make a world record, but his father's affidavit is very elaborate. Of course, Tom may be disappointed if his feat isn't counted,*" *his mother said.*

Already, however, Mrs. Andrews said her son is looking for another record to destroy. He may try the omelets after all.

HOMAGE TO JOE BRAINARD

Hours *in codeine's loose grip.*

Morning. As I waited for Carrie's daily visit, trying to catch some sleep but unable to, a tape loop of "Laurel and Hardy: An Oral Hystery" kept running through my inner ear, spliced and patched with the strict evangelical warnings John gave me toward the end of his life.

There was John's liveliest voice, the voice of "Babe" Hardy, robust and ebullient. That voice I could respond to, interact with:

> INTERVIEWER: Babe, in your mind, what was the single funniest sound effect you and Stan created?
>
> HARDY: In *The Perfect Day* I hit Stan on the head with an automobile jack, and the blow sounded like the ringing of an anvil when struck with a twelve-pound hammer.
>
> LAUREL: I remember being jealous that I never got to hit Ollie with an automobile jack. It looked like terrific fun.

And here was John's late voice, his last voice as it turned out, the voice of a TV desert prophet, earnest and humorless and alone:

You have only as much of Jesus in you as you have the spirit of obedience. Evangelism is one beggar telling another beggar where to find bread. When you study the scriptures "hit or miss," you're likely to miss more than you hit.

The voices competed for my assent. They plagued my ears like cicadas.

INTERVIEWER: Stan, you probably fell down more flights of stairs than anyone in screen history.

LAUREL: I never thought there was anything funny about a guy falling down the stairs.

HARDY: I did.

The flower of self-respect cannot grow in the soil of sinful habit. We must adjust to the Bible—never the Bible to ourselves.

INTERVIEWER: I remember seeing a picture with a goat.

HARDY: How dare you? Insulting Stan like that. My word.

LAUREL: Very funny, Babe.

INTERVIEWER: No, a real goat. It followed you around through the whole film.

LAUREL: Right. That was *Angora Love*. It had no plot, really. Just that goat—but we sure got a lot of footage out of him. I give a piece of cookie to the goat and he wants more, so he follows us around. We try every conceivable way to get rid of him, but no use. We hid, we walked backward, we disguised ourselves. Nothing helped.

Salvation is free, but it costs you an enormous price. Failure is the path of least persistence.

HARDY: We finally brought the goat to our room because the word had spread that a goat had been
stolen and we didn't want to be arrested as goat-
nappers. The comedy in our room consisted
mainly of the goat eating the stuffing from the fur-
niture and my pants. It was very simple.

*Never try to bear tomorrow's burden with today's grace. A
truth not practiced is a truth not believed.*

INTERVIEWER: Now, Stan, tell us how you developed
your famous cry.
LAUREL: Well, the funny thing about that cry is, it's the
only mannerism I ever used in the films that I
didn't like. When we would be improvising something on the set and we came to a pause where we
couldn't think of anything to do, Roach always insisted that I use the cry. It always got a laugh, and
it sure became part of my standard equipment,
but somehow I never had any affection for it.

*The Bible has survived the ignorance of its friends and the
hatred of its enemies. God may lead you around, but He will
always lead you aright.*

—————

The voices were part of an internal pressure that presaged
and accompanied a piece of writing about John. It had been
nine years since his death. During that time I had taken up
many times—in poems, stories, plays, essays—the Sisyphean
task of inserting him back into reality. "When someone you
love dies," Mark Twain wrote, "it is like when your house
burns down; it isn't for years that you realize the extent of

your loss." From my hygienic room in the hospital, I could hear the burning house collapsing. I could smell the acrid odor of black smoke.

I relied on a familiar exercise to help aerate the burning house. In 1985 I ran across Joe Brainard's extraordinary books *I Remember* and *More I Remember* in the stacks at the University of Virginia's Alderman Library. Brainard's books are composed entirely of short recollections, each beginning with the words *I remember* . . . :

> *I remember the first time I got a letter that said "After Five Days Return To" on the envelope, and I thought that after I had kept the letter for five days I was supposed to return it to the sender.*

> *I remember when, in high school, if you wore green and yellow on Thursday it meant that you were queer.*

> *I remember monkeys who did modern paintings and won prizes.*

Brainard offers a simple and direct way to sort through memories, affections, chronic angers, and so forth. The directness and simplicity are profound blessings. I often resorted to Brainard's "I remember" format when I felt at a far distance from language, for whatever reason. Now that I was close to the end of a dose of codeine, I wrote a few Brainard-like recollections before my consciousness rejected everything but the nerve endings in my right leg. Imitating Brainard's short, declarative sentences was like reaching out for a well-anchored lifeline.

> *I remember John throwing away his Led Zeppelin albums because they were not "of the Lord."*

I remember the first time I saw the pink surgical scars crisscrossing the tender pulp of John's abdomen.

I remember the shock of running into John and his high school buddies drinking beer behind the local swimming pool. "Look at Mini-Brute chug it!" someone called out when John drank. I wondered if he'd have to undergo an extra run on dialysis.

I remember John on dialysis holding his penis tenderly and nonsexually. Sometimes my father would say, "For God's sake, get your hand out of your pants!"

I remember that once he passed puberty, John was never without a beard.

I remember practicing for hours to learn Jimi Hendrix's solos and riffs in "Purple Haze." When it came on the radio one day, I casually played along with Jimi. John was amazed. "You did it! You got it right!" he said. Then: "How'd you do that?"

I remember asking John who was the greatest writer who ever lived. He said Shakespeare. When I asked him why, he said, "Because he probably gives you the best account of what it's like to be alive."

I remember John learning German so he could correspond with German stamp collectors.

I remember that the last movie I saw with John was Monty Python's Life of Brian. He thought it was funny but blasphemous. I thought it was funny and respectful of Christ. "It's about a guy who gets confused for Christ," I argued. "They weren't saying

Brian was Christ." "Maybe so," John said, "but something's not right about it, even though I laughed."

I remember our running into Bob Long's Hobby Shop. We headed straight for the HO car track. Anyone could use the track, but you had to bring your own car. I remember being too shy to race with the other kids, while John stepped right into the fray.

I remember wondering if John would ever get married.

I remember that the hair around John's shunt (in his right arm) was forever being shaved, and how the shaved spot looked like a woman's underarm.

I remember John refusing to eat Quisp cereal. Quisp was my cereal. John ate Frosted Flakes and Rice Krispies.

I remember days when John was so disoriented, he couldn't speak.

I remember the wallpaper John picked out after Dad said he could have any type he wanted. It was printed with black-and-white squares in a twisting, psychedelic pattern. The first week after it was up, I thought I was going to get seasick just standing in the room.

I remember watching John pray in his room. He'd kneel beside his bed, knees on the bare wood floor. I'd watch from my room down the hall, my door open just a hair.

I remember our making fun of Dad's multihour slide shows.

I remember that John went to a sensitivity workshop and had his umbrella stolen.

GUINNESS SUPERLATIVES LIMITED
2 Cecil Court, London Road
Enfield, Middlesex EN2 6DJ
Telephone: 01 366 4551
Telegrams and cables: Mostest Enfield

Mr H Raymond Andrews Jr
1714 Rolling Hills Circle
Charleston
West Virginia 25314
USA

19 February 1973

Dear Mr Andrews:

Mr David Boehm, President of the Sterling Publishing Company, brought across your correspondence on his visit to London earlier this month.

As you can appreciate when dealing with records of the unofficial kind such as hand clapping, we have to work on a basis of comparability. In the matter of the rate and of the audible range, we would not, in this instance, be comparing like with like.

I am prepared to accept the variation in rate because it is disposed that your son did not allow the rate to drop below one hundred claps per minute. The only difficulty is now the question of the audible range. His feat of stamina was performed indoors, whereas the existing record was performed outdoors.

I would ask you to carry out a test to see at what range clapping of the same average figure as he was able to maintain during the fourteen-plus hours would in fact be audible in windless conditions out of doors in a field in which there were no surrounding echoing surfaces.

Perhaps you would be good enough to write me on this point so that we can make a final decision on this matter.

With all best wishes.

Yours sincerely,
NORRIS D McWHIRTER
Editor

THIRTEEN WAYS OF LOOKING
AT MY MOTHER AND FATHER

But there's no vocabulary
For love within a family, love that's lived in
But not looked at, love within the light of which
All else is seen, the love within which
All other love finds speech.
This love is silent.

— T. S. ELIOT

I.

My mother and father arrived from Grand Rapids, emissaries from the mysterious sunlit world. It was midmorning. Carrie had called them and forgotten to tell me. Their arrival took me completely by surprise.

I am not gifted with an unusually keen sense of smell. But the first sight of my mother and father walking through the door to my hospital room attached itself with peculiar force to the hospital's vinegary, dustless odor; and I was delivered instantly back to the fourth floor of St. Mary's Hospital in Grand Rapids.

———

March 23, 1980. My mother and father and I are walking down a long hallway toward John's room. John was admitted three days ago. His white blood cell count was up, he felt nauseous, he couldn't stop coughing. Whatever he had, he couldn't shake it. A month earlier he had been living in Lexington, taking classes at the University of Kentucky in between runs on dialysis, when he collapsed on the stairs to his dormitory. A janitor found him in a heap and carried him to his room. John's doctor in Lexington, a steamroller whom John suffered the way he suffered endless injections of heparin, set up an appointment for John with a neurologist. But the earliest the neurologist could see John was in six days.

John fell again the next day. His legs simply stopped working. This time a fellow student carried him to his room. Later that night John discovered he could use only the muscles in his neck and face. Otherwise, he was paralyzed. He was having trouble breathing. The head resident of his dormitory called an ambulance, then our house in Grand Rapids. My mother spoke with the doctor at the emergency room. "I looked at the backs of his eyes," the emergency-room doctor told my mother. "They were like an eighty-year-old's."

My mother and father and I drove to Lexington immediately, anxious and confused.

John pulled through. By the time we got to the University of Kentucky Hospital, his muscle control had returned as capriciously as it had departed. He was walking around his room and chatting with the nurses, all of whom adored him. He wanted to go back to classes.

"Don't rush it," my mother said. "The Lord wants you to make sure you're well, He's with you."

"I know He is," John said, a little annoyed at being lectured. "But I'm not much use to Him here."

"Oh yes you are," my mother said, determination rising in her. "You never know how the Lord's using you. Could be the guy in the next room needs to see your cheerfulness to get through the day."

"I don't always feel so cheerful," John said weakly.

"There's always prayer," my mother said. "The Lord's right here by you all the time."

"I know," John said. "I know."

I never entered into these discussions of the Lord's will if I could help it. It would only upset my mother and father. My father kept silent, watching TV or reading the paper, but he was like a wind sock, registering any disagreements that rippled through the room's air. Sensing disagreement, he would look up disapprovingly and say, "That's enough of that. That won't help anybody."

So my father and I watched a basketball game on TV while John and my mother discussed the Lord's desire for cheerful followers. LSU was playing Kentucky in the SEC championship game. I was astonished at how effectively my father could concentrate on the game. I couldn't. Rage made me sullen. I wanted to erupt, shout out, "Leave John alone! He's sick! The Lord doesn't give a shit about his cheerfulness!"

But I didn't. I sat in my chair, fuming, wishing I were somewhere else — or wishing I were able to spend some time alone with John.

When LSU won the game by two points, my father said to John, who hadn't paid the least bit of attention to the game, "What a shame. I'm sorry your team lost." Then my father and mother and I went back to the hotel.

After three weeks in the University of Kentucky Hospital, unable to shake whatever virus he had, John flew home to Grand Rapids. A week later he was admitted to St. Mary's Hospital, fighting the same virus. Running on dialysis, he felt nauseous, and his temperature leveled off at 102.5. His white blood cell count shot up again. He kept coughing, deep hacking outbursts.

This time, to everyone's relief, John did not lose the use of his legs or of any muscles. One day he wanted to walk to the hospital gift shop to get a book of crossword puzzles. I said I'd go with him.

"Okay," my mother said reluctantly. "But don't dally. And don't go ahead of him. Stay right with him."

"Of course," I said, feeling the familiar rage build in me. "You think I'd leave him somewhere?"

"Drop it," John whispered to me. He knew that the conversation, if pursued, would make us all regretful. He was right. I said to my mother, "We'll be fine. Don't worry. I'll stay right with him."

"How's your job going?" John asked with effort as we walked out into the hallway.

"It's incredibly boring," I said. I was working at a clothing store in the big mall on Twenty-eighth Street in Grand Rapids. "I'm really glad I'm not there today."

As soon as I said it, I felt a rush of shame. "I mean, not that I'm glad to be *here*," I said.

"It's okay," John said, reassuring me. "I know what you mean."

John looked back to his room. He was determining whether we were safely out of earshot of my mother and father.

"Playing guitar with anybody?" he asked nonchalantly, still looking back at the room. Before I had a chance to answer, he stopped walking and grabbed my hand. He looked at me, his eyes radiant with candor, and said, "You've got to respect your mother and father. The Bible's clear about that."

John started down the hallway again, this time with difficulty. He was staggering and having trouble breathing.

"I think we've gone far enough," I said, trying not to panic. John looked as though he couldn't take another step.

"Get a wheelchair," John said. "My legs are killing me."

A folded-up wheelchair was right beside us in the hallway. I unfolded it, secured the locks, and helped John sit down. "Let's go back to the room," I said. It was the last place I wanted to go, but I was scared.

"Yes," John said.

I wheeled John back to the room. My mother and father met us, their eyes wide with alarm. I waited for my mother to ask me if I had done something to provoke John's attack of breathlessness and fatigue. When she didn't ask, I felt guilty for expecting her to.

"I'm just tired," John said, objecting to the fuss we were making over him. "I just need to lie down."

John went to sleep immediately. The doctor on call, whom my mother had summoned, walked in a while later and woke up John with his stethoscope. "How are you feeling?" the doctor asked as he poked and prodded. He was a large, tense man with no hair.

"Tired," John said.

The doctor took John's temperature and blood pressure and looked into his eyes. John's temperature was up again; his blood pressure was fine. My mother engaged the doctor in conversation, asked the right questions, presented a robust, courageous face. She was very good with doctors. It was a skill she had honed over the years. My father and I said nothing.

Again John showed every sign of pulling through. His temperature dropped, his coughing abated. At the end of visiting hours, we went home feeling reassured that John was going to be all right. He had a virus of some kind, the doctor had said, much like a cold. And while prednisone (a steroid that John took initially to prevent his body from rejecting his transplanted kidney and that he continued to take when he was back on dialysis to help his body retain proteins otherwise lost in his urine) made any virus potentially dangerous, as it increased his susceptibility to infection, John'd been confronted with worse episodes before and come through.

"Still," the doctor said, "let's keep him here where we can keep an eye on him."

It is now ten o'clock the next morning and my mother and father and I are walking down the hallway of the fourth floor toward John's room, the dustless, vinegary smell assaulting us. Twenty minutes earlier we'd received a phone call from the nurses' station, the anonymous voice telling us to come to the hospital at once. I knew immediately what had happened. I said nothing.

Seeing us approach John's room, the head nurse plants herself in front of us as though she is setting a pick in a basketball game and tells us to wait in a private consultation room, where the doctor wants to meet with us.

"Why can't I see my son?" my mother asks. She says it curtly, without emotion, as if that will persuade the nurse to let her go straight to John. "Where is my son?" Fury lurks under the taut surface of her voice. The head nurse doesn't budge.

My father doesn't speak. I can't. My legs take me to the consultation room. As soon as we sit down, the door opens. It is the tense bald doctor.

John's heart stopped an hour ago. The tense doctor's lips move, absurd noises issuing from his throat like smoke. At some point I understand he's speaking words. He couldn't restart John's heart. Did he say *jump start?* I see two crumpled junkers nose to nose, jumper cables running between them like tentacles in bright confusion.

John is dead.

The tense doctor acquired speech in order to tell us this: John is dead.

John's death is now a fact vying among other facts. But there are no other facts.

The chaplain arrives. Noises issue from his throat. He leads us to John's room. My legs follow.

John lies on the bed, the covers pulled up to his neck. He looks peaceful, as the chaplain said he would look, but too artfully arranged, as though he's already at the funeral home. All signs of this morning's struggle have been fastidiously concealed. My mother breaks away from my father, whose arm had been around her shoulder, and grabs John's hand and wails. "*Won't you come back*," she demands, her lips burrowing into his hand, her wail a rip in the room's stillness, her ache as old as language. "*Won't you come back*."

My father and I stare wordlessly, as though over the edge of a cliff. I see very clearly the lineaments of my brother's face. I see the coarse black beard he never shaved. I see the cheeks made puffy by prednisone. I see the waxy, pale skin shining under the harsh light.

John's body is hiding something, withholding a secret. I want desperately to be in on it.

I look around the room. Is John now in one of the high corners, abstract as mathematics and just as self-aware, a sleight-of-hand shadow, a hovering spectator emptied of himself, looking down at us?

I stare and stare into the corners of the room, the whitewashed ceiling and walls, the immaculate floor. I see nothing.

I look at my mother and father.

I have never seen them before.

2.

"How you feeling?" my father asked as my mother hugged me. "We thought about coming last night, but the snow scared us." My father held a vase of tulips. "Where should I . . . I'll put these here, where you can see them." He set the tulips down on the thin rollaway table I'd been writing on.

"Hi, hi," I said. "Oh, look at those. Thanks."

"We're just as sorry as we could be," my mother said. "I hate to see you like this." I hadn't noticed before that she was carrying a paper bag.

"Thanks, Mom, Dad. Thanks for coming. I hope your drive over went okay."

"It was fine," my father said. "I'm afraid we would have had trouble if we'd come last night."

"Of course," I said. "It's good you didn't try to drive over in the snow. Have a seat. Do you want to sit down? I'm sure we could rustle up another chair."

"No," my mother said. "I'm tired of sitting. It feels good to stand."

"I'd rather stand," my father said.

"Here's something for you," my mother said, handing me an envelope that I assumed contained a get-well card.

"You didn't need to do that," I said, opening the envelope and pulling out the card. The card featured a photograph of a windmill surrounded by red and yellow tulips. Inside the card, the words *Hope You're Feeling Better Soon!* were printed in an elaborately serifed script. Below the script was a note in my mother's handwriting:

> *Jesus says, I am the resurrection and the life. He who believes in Me shall live even if he dies, and everyone who lives and believes in Me shall never die.*
>
> *Love, Mom & Dad*

I thought about making a joke to the effect that, by the most anal retentive of grammatical rules, it was uncertain whether the *Me* in the second sentence referred to Christ or to Mom and Dad. But even I didn't want to make such a smart-ass remark.

"Thanks," I said.

"You're welcome," my mother said, digging into the paper bag she'd been carrying. "We brought you some things that might make the time go by faster. Remember this?"

Out of the bag she lifted an old scrapbook containing newspaper clippings and letters generated by my breaking the world record for clapping in 1972. I hadn't looked at it in years. "Look at that old thing!" I said. "Jeez, I'd forgotten all about it."

"*And,*" my mother said, pausing for dramatic effect, "I thought this might be fun to look at." This time she pulled out a photo album. Every year since 1954 my father had made our family's Christmas card, based on one of his own photographs. My mother had brought an album containing every card he had made since 1954.

"Great," I said. "I can't wait to show this to Carrie."

"Is Carrie at work?" my mother said.

"She's teaching her computer graphics course," I said. "She'll be here this afternoon."

My father took the photo album out of my mother's hands and opened it to the Christmas card he had made for 1972. "Let's see," he said. "You broke the clapping record in seventy-two. Remember this one?" He handed me the album opened to an image of John running on dialysis.

What, I wondered, did my parents' friends think upon receiving this image of holiday cheer? John is "life size" while my father and mother and I are lilliputian, dwarfed by John and especially by the dialysis machine. I hang glee-fully from a scissor clamp—a scissor clamp, I noticed, that is directing the flow of John's blood into the machine. My mother sits sidesaddle on the deck of the machine, beaming as though Elvis were about to appear any second (no, with those glasses, she's waiting for Buddy Holly), and my

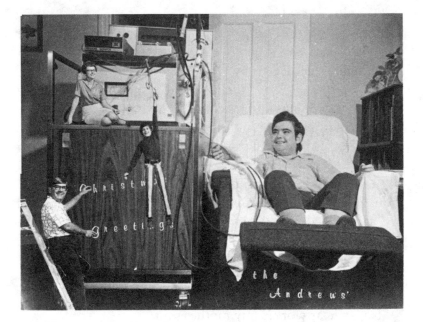

father has pitched a stepladder beside the machine and is lining up the letters *h* and *G* in *Christmas Greetings*. John looks with immense satisfaction at his blood as it travels through tubes leading from his shunt to the machine and back again.

"I think this one's my favorite," I said. "Of them all, I'm pretty sure it's my favorite."

"Thank you," my father said.

"It's brilliant," my mother said proudly, patting my father on the back. "Just like your father."

"I love the way the dialysis machine looms over us," I said. "The way it did in our lives. But I have to wonder what your friends thought when they got it in the mail."

My father tilted his head. He seemed surprised that anyone would ask such a question. "It's a happy picture," he said as though it were the most obvious thing in the world. "It says that we were a happy family, even though we had challenges to face. People understood it to be a picture of hope."

"But," I said, "the image is so wonderfully *weird*. I mean, look at it. Sure, there's hopefulness in it. But there are all kinds of frustrations there, too. Confusions, frustrations. Don't you think?"

"No," my father said. "It's a *happy* picture. We're *smiling*. See? And people responded to it that way."

"But don't you like the idea that the picture is rich enough—"

"That *is* the way people responded," my father said. "They saw it as a happy picture."

"I was just thinking—"

"I told you how they responded. How many times do I have to say it?"

"Why don't we look at this later," my mother said, taking the album.

3.

My parents must have felt that I was emotionally blackmailing them. Obviously they needed to spend most of their time with John. I understood that. I even preferred it. But my mother and father tortured themselves, I think, over what they saw as their neglecting me. I tried to make them understand, carefully, without upsetting them, that I didn't *want* them to spend more time with me. I was living out a dream scenario for a hemophiliac. My parents weren't hovering over my every move. For long periods of time I was unaccounted for, and I loved it. Conflicting desire was like a spy in the house. On the one hand, my parents wanted assurance that God and others thought it was all right that they let their hemophiliac son compete in skateboard competitions, play in a punk band, hang out with "questionable" characters. On the other hand, they wanted assurance that I needed them — or, at least, that I wanted more of their care than they could give me. And that latter assurance I was unable to give.

4.

Here is a story my mother tells frequently and with great good humor. In 1968 my mother and father met with a nephrologist at Columbus Children's Hospital. The nephrologist sat on the other side of a gorgeous cherry desk.

"I'm sorry," the nephrologist began. "The dye tests we ran through John's system confirm that he has kidney disease."

Silence.

"What's a kidney?" my mother asked.

With each retelling, my father seems pained in a new way.

5.

My mother and father looked at my bleeding gums and shook their heads. "Maybe you're using too much elbow grease?" my father said. I didn't understand the question. I couldn't make my inept dry elbows secrete a thing; I'd tried. My mother handed me a new orange toothbrush and pointed to the bathroom. "This time," she said, "don't put so much elbow grease into it. Take it easy on yourself."

6.

One Saturday afternoon my mother and father met me in the backyard. I'd just ridden my Suzuki home from practicing at the makeshift motocross track my friends and I had constructed at a nearby chicken farm.

My father tried to speak over the sound of the Suzuki. "I saw all those — "

I shook my head to let him know I couldn't hear him until the bike's motor quit. I took off my helmet, and we waited wordlessly for the bike to stop coughing.

"I saw your grades," my father began. "And I saw all those motorcycle magazines in your room. I know you're trying to get bad grades because you want to imitate the losers in those magazines."

My mother didn't say anything, but her presence implied moral support of my father.

"That's not true," I said. "Those guys are smart. You don't — "

"Don't interrupt me when I'm talking to you," my father said. "You're *trying* to look dumb so you'll fit in with that crowd you're hanging out with."

"Who's dumb? David? Tommy?"

"I told you not to interrupt. Now put the bike away and get cleaned up for dinner."

Later that night, my father said, "You know, if John weren't on dialysis, we wouldn't let you have a motorcycle."

It fell like a thunderclap: the knowledge that my parents harbored untold guilt over John and me, as if they had willfully inflicted our diseases upon us. The power of that knowledge made me tremble. The power was appalling. Like Toto in *The Wizard of Oz,* I had peeked behind the wizard's curtain and seen a desperate man — and woman — improvising at the controls.

7.

"I don't think I can talk anymore," I said.

"That's fine," my mother said.

"I know how you feel," my father said.

I looked at Carrie.

"Why don't we go get a cup of coffee," Carrie said.

8.

Several times during my marathon conversation with Ellen, she interrupted me to say, "Tom, Tom, Tom, your parents were saints!"

9.

I decided to give the Christmas card album another try. I turned to the image my father made for 1975.

"I like the puzzle quality of this one," I said.

My mother looked over my shoulder at the image. "Nineteen seventy-five," she said. "That's the year John got his transplant at the Cleveland Clinic. We were there for — what? Four months?"

"Four months," my father said. "Four very long months."

"Oh," my mother said. "I had that pseudo-gout. Remember? I was in a wheelchair and you wheeled me across Euclid Avenue to the hotel through a *terrible* blizzard. I'll never forget it."

"That's right," my father said. "The Park Plaza Hotel. It was a certifiable blizzard."

"I'll never forget the doctor I talked to on the phone," my mother said. "He called and said they had a kidney for John — "

"They got it," my father interrupted, "from a twenty-four-year-old man who'd been shot in the head. In a bar in Akron."

"I asked him about the operation," my mother continued, "and he said 'Zee plumbing eez zimple.'"

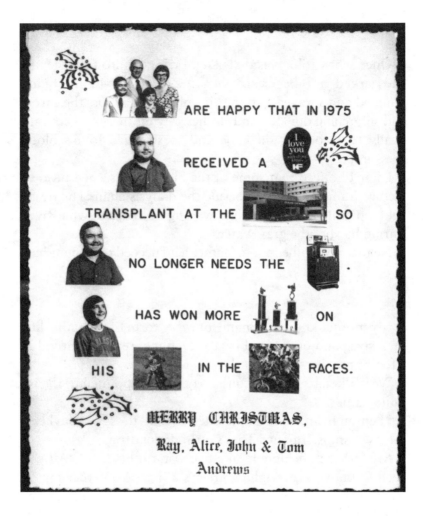

ARE HAPPY THAT IN 1975

RECEIVED A

TRANSPLANT AT THE SO

NO LONGER NEEDS THE .

HAS WON MORE ON

HIS IN THE RACES.

MERRY CHRISTMAS,

Ray, Alice, John & Tom

Andrews

My mother grinned widely. I'd never heard her imitate a voice before. She was good at it!

"I didn't know Colonel Klink performed the transplant," I said.

My mother and father laughed, and I was grateful.

10.

Once when John was dialyzing, I tripped into the machine and jerked a tube clean out of its socket. John's blood pumped and sprayed into the air, splattering across the carpet and splotching our skin and clothes. My mother worked frantically to reconnect the tube and to stabilize John's blood pressure.

Later I noticed that some of the blood had seeped inside a picture frame on the wall beside the dialysis chair. The frame held a picture of John and me wading in the Kanawha River, staring hard at the gray water.

Neither my mother nor my father felt I needed to be punished.

11.

My mother knows the name of every form of vegetable life, each sprig and bud. She'd try to teach me, recalcitrant kid in a fog of numbers and wheels.

We walked beside the house. My mother pointed to the infinite names.

"Lemon balm," she said. "Smell it? And those are daylilies. That's cosmos. Yarrow. That's a rhododendron."

My father interrupted, an elfish grin on his face. "All you need to know is, everything green's a lilac. My father taught me that. Every week he'd say he was going out to mow the lilacs."

12.

In the summer of 1985 my mother and father gave a poetry reading. They didn't tell me about it until two weeks afterward. By then, my mother said, maybe I wouldn't be upset.

I had been invited to give a reading at the Grand Rapids City Arts Festival. Carrie and I were living in Charlottesville, Virginia, waiting for graduate school to start in the fall and in the interim exploring employment opportunities as a bank teller and as a clerk at 7-Eleven, respectively. We couldn't afford a trip to Grand Rapids, and the Arts Festival offered no honorarium. I'd been to the Arts Festival readings before. They were pleasant enough events but not worth giving up three days of work.

My mother and father felt differently. One shouldn't turn down such invitations, they argued, because of the vital networking that goes on.

"Networking? What networking?" I said on the phone to my mother. "Usually there are only about six people in the audience. And three of them are hoping the event has something to do with poultry."

"Doesn't matter how many people show up," my mother said. "What matters is the one contact who might be able to help you get a teaching job."

"You have a point, theoretically," I said. "But the odds are astronomical."

"So you're not coming," my mother said. "That's your decision."

"Right," I said. "I'm sorry. I'm not coming."

Two weeks later my mother and father called with, as my father put it, "some rather . . . interesting news. Our poetry reading went very well."

"Your *what?*" I said.

"Now, don't get mad," my mother said. She was on the cordless phone in their bedroom. It crackled and hissed through her words. "We just couldn't live with the idea of your passing up the contacts you'd make at that festival reading."

"Oh, my God," I said. I felt dizzy.

"So we went and read your poems for you," my father said. "And if I do say so myself, we did your poems proud."

"You should've heard your father," my mother said. "He had them roaring. He's so witty."

"And your mother did an excellent job," my father said. "Just excellent."

"I surprised myself," my mother said. "I didn't understand a word I read, but that didn't seem to matter."

I was speechless.

"How many people were in the audience?" I asked. It seemed as good a question as any.

"Oh, about twenty," my father said. "Wouldn't you say?"

"At least twenty," my mother said. "More like thirty, I'd say."

I tried to imagine the two of them standing in front of thirty people reading my poems. An image festered and grew in my mind of an audience full of my favorite contemporary poets. Jean Valentine, Charles Wright, Yehuda Amichai, Michael Palmer — I watched one poet after another enter the room in a boisterous procession, eventually quieting down to hear my mother and father read my poems. I was mortified.

"What was that all about?" Carrie asked when I hung up the phone. "You look white as a sheet."

"I need a drink," I said.

————

The longer I thought about my parents' reading, however, the more the idea charmed me. Yes, their action was a shining example of "unrespected boundaries," as psychotherapists put it. (Respecting boundaries seems to be, from my experience and observation, one of the harder lessons for parents of chronically ill children to learn.) That made me furious. But otherwise, what was their crime? So my parents were oblivious to the rules of the literary world; so what? Now they knew the rules. I decided it was worth suffering (once!) the mortification I felt, if only to carry to the grave an image of my father's reading, in his supremely rational reading voice, "Dr. Farnsworth, a Chiropodist, Lived in Ohio, Where He Wrote Only the First Lines of Poems," a poem I'd written out of a Monty Python poetic:

1.

The moon smells like a fishbone. The cow

2.

Plotinus, Porphory, strolling the lake's

3.

1925. *Mountain, Table, Anchors, Navel*

4.

The smell of God in wood.

5.

"She came to him, nuzzling his chest."

6.

Chaos in ochre. Time in the physical. Light

7.

Past the barn, past the worm-ridden apple trees

8.

Organ swell. Cadence. Swedenborg with a walk-
    ing stick,

9.

The sun, lost

10.

I have never dreamed of water.

11.

Will God work only in Geometry, Emerson

12.

Say of me that I am living still.

—and of my mother reading an elegy I'd written called "Paul Celan":

You've fingered your death
like a bread crumb in your pocket.
You're taking it

out. You're placing it on your lip.

Are you asleep?
—There's No-one's voice again.

13.

We were driving through the desert in a VW camper. We passed prickly pear cacti, tumbleweed, earth tiered into seven or eight different shades of red. We drove toward black pools in the road that turned out to be nothing. My father was at the wheel. My mother studied the road map on her lap. John had been asleep for hours in the back of the camper.

I sat on a cushion just behind the driver's seat, acting cool in my new sunglasses.

"Peace," I said, holding up two fingers.

"We're coming up on Flagstaff," my mother said.

"Where's that?" I said.

"Still Arizona," my mother said.

We drove and drove.

"How old are you?" my father said.

"Me? Nine," I said.

"Shame on you," he said. "When I was your age, I was eleven."

I squealed with pleasure.

National Enquirer   September 9, 1973

DIRECTOR WHO MADE "SOUTH PACIFIC" REVEALS HE WAS
MENTALLY ILL FOR 28 YEARS

TWINS ENGAGED, MARRIED AND HAVE BABY ON SAME DAY

SMOTHERING SNEEZES CAN HARM YOU, WARNS DOCTOR

11-YEAR-OLD BOY CLAPS 94,520 TIMES IN
14 HOURS 31 MINUTES

Tom Andrews doesn't expect anybody to give him a hand for breaking a world's record. Especially after clapping for himself an astounding 94,520 times!

"I just wanted to break a world's record," grinned freckle-faced Tom, who lives with his parents in Charleston, W.Va.

Norris McWhirter, co-compiler of the Guinness Book, *told the* Enquirer: *"We don't have many 11-year-olds in the* Guinness Book. *So this is quite a remarkable feat."*

SIGNS ARE TAKEN FOR WONDERS

That your scrapbook?" Ellen asked.

I was writing in my notebook with one hand and paging through the scrapbook of newspaper clippings and letters my mother had brought me with the other.

It was the end of the week. My leg had stopped leaking fresh blood into the knee, calf, and ankle. The pain, unmedicated, was still outrageous — and would remain so until my body had a chance to loosen and break down and absorb the hardened blood inside the leg. But the emergency had passed. All I could do was wait, and I could do that at home. My hematologist said we should wait one more day before putting a cast on my broken ankle; then I could go home.

When I muttered to Ellen that, technically, the scrapbook belonged to my mother, who had brought it to the hospital to cheer me up, Ellen glanced at the *National Enquirer* headline with my picture beneath it and said, "You did that? Clapped your hands?"

I nodded.

"Lord!" she said. "Did you have a major bleed, or what?"

I shook my head. "You'd think so, but I didn't," I said. "It was the strangest thing. My hands weren't sore at all. I could have gone on another couple of hours at least."

Just then I had the pleasant and somewhat disorienting experience of bringing to mind something I'd never recalled before: the very moment, about two hours into the clapping, when I realized how easy it was going to be to keep a precise, consistent rhythm. That was the moment I knew I would break the record. It was going to be a piece of cake. My hands, like the legs of runners who have broken through the "wall," hammered away at themselves effortlessly and indefinitely. Hammered.

I hadn't yet been diagnosed with hemophilia, but I'd experienced enough bleeds in my knees, ankles, elbows, fingers, and toes to recognize the telltale signs that foreshadowed them: the tingling sensation inside the joint, the warmth of the skin and muscles. I felt no trace of those signs while I clapped. I was confident I would not start a bleed, even though at that point I didn't know what my bleeds meant — or even to call them "bleeds." ("Deep bruises," we called them.) Back then I thought I was no different from other children, only clumsier, more accident-prone. I thought all healthy kids bled into their joints the way I did. John never experienced a joint or muscle bleed, but he wasn't able to play outside.

"How long did you clap?" Ellen asked as she scanned the *National Enquirer* article.

"Um, fourteen hours and thirty-one minutes," I said.

"And you're telling me your hands didn't hurt at all?"

"It's true," I said. "Believe me, you could do it if you wanted to."

"No no no no," Ellen said, grinning. "Nothing could get me to clap that long. Did your record ever get broken?"

"The next year somebody clapped something like sixteen hours. Now the record is around sixty hours. It's incredible. Somewhere in there, fifty-eight, fifty-nine. Some guy in India clapped that long."

Ellen took a look at my ankle. "Look at those colors," she said.

"I know," I said. "It used to be the color of an iris but now it looks more like bright rust."

"I don't think I've ever met anybody who's been in the *Guinness Book of World Records* before," Ellen said. "Or the *National Enquirer*. Was this on a Sunday?"

"Actually it was a Wednesday. But it was a parent–teacher conference day, so there was no school. I could've gone longer, but my parents made me go to bed."

Ellen said, "But by then you'd broken the record, so it didn't matter, right?"

"Exactly," I said. "Once I broke the record, I was ready to try something else. I was thinking about cooking more than seventy-five omelettes in half an hour."

"Your poor mother," Ellen said, shaking her head. Then: "It's some story you got there. Ever written about it?"

AFFIDAVIT

STATE OF WEST VIRGINIA
COUNTY OF KANAWHA, TO WIT:

LEONARD SARGEANT III, of 1726 Rolling Hills Circle, Charleston, Kanawha County, West Virginia 25314, being first duly sworn upon his oath deposes and says that he is forty-two (42) years of age; that he is a neighbor and personal acquaintance of Thomas C. Andrews, who resides at 1714 Rolling Hills Circle; that on the 15th day of November, 1972, he visited the residence of said Thomas C. Andrews, at which time he saw and heard said Thomas C. Andrews in the act of continuous hand-clapping; that on Saturday, March 24, 1973, at approximately 1:30 in the afternoon he accompanied said Thomas C. Andrews to the athletic field of John Adams Junior High School, located in a remote area in the city of Charleston, West Virginia; that he and said Thomas C. Andrews stood at opposite football goalposts one hundred and twenty (120) yards apart; that said Thomas C. Andrews commenced clapping his hands in the same manner observed by him on the 15th day of November, 1972; that said hand-clapping was clearly audible; that there were no surrounding echoing surfaces; and that at the time of said hand-clapping he was standing upwind of said Thomas C. Andrews in a very light breeze adverse to the audibility of said hand-clapping.

Dated this 27th day of March, 1973.

LEONARD SARGEANT III

Taken, sworn to, and acknowledged before me, a Notary Public in and for the county and state aforesaid, this 27th day of March, 1973.

*Given under my hand and notarial seal this 27th day of
March, 1973.*
My commision expires January 21, 1974.

MAE U. ADAMS
Notary Public, Kanawha County,
West Virginia

PART THREE

On Being a
Bad Insurance Risk

The National Tattler   January 23, 1973

BOY BREAKS HAND-CLAPPING RECORD
HE PROBABLY NEVER WILL APPLAUD ANYONE!

ON BEING A BAD INSURANCE RISK

1. On Being a Bad Insurance Risk

"How well one has to be, to be ill!" wrote Alice James in her diary. That paradoxical remark gets at the heart of what I hope this book is about. Negotiating hemophilia, for me, has meant finding strategies to be well — or to approach being well — while in the midst of significant upheaval and danger "to life and limb," as the saying goes. When I was growing up in Charleston, West Virginia, my strategies were aggressively unconventional. I raced motorcycles, competed in skateboard contests, joined a punk rock band, even (when I was eleven, before I was officially diagnosed with hemophilia) broke the world record for handclapping, which landed me in *The Guinness Book of World Records*.

Looking back, I realize I was trying to deny at all costs the received image of hemophilia — or of any chronic illness. Hemophiliacs, that image suggests, must lead a silent, sedentary life; must follow doctors' orders with exemplary, even saintly, resignation; must *look and act sick*. My brother's response to kidney disease was to live out just such an image. Perhaps I was staking a claim to my own experience of illness, apart from my brother's. Or perhaps I simply liked the idea of being a bad insurance risk.

Hearing even these few facts about my life, people often ask me, "Motorcycle racing? Competitive skateboarding? How could your parents allow it? What were they *thinking*?"

As I mentioned earlier, my brother's illness was worse than mine and demanded more time and care. The exigencies of the home dialysis patient are unimaginably stressful and demanding. My problems diminished in comparison because they were intermittent: bleeds didn't occur every day, or every other day like John's dialysis. As a result, I was the healthy child in the house. It was an auspicious designation. It meant I could prowl the streets with neighborhood kids, get into the usual trouble, even participate in the more extravagant activities I've mentioned.

It's also true that though I suffered many severe bleeds throughout my childhood, I was not diagnosed with hemophilia until I was fifteen. Before then, our family doctor would throw up his hands at my repeated bleeding and mutter something like "It's the darnedest thing" before aspirating the blood from my flushed knee or ankle with a syringe the size of a small Buick. Aspiration, my hematologist at the University of Michigan Hospital told me years later, was precisely the wrong course of action. It simply creates more room inside the joint for blood to rush into and fill. "It's a miracle," my hematologist said, "that you're not permanently crippled. The cartilage in your joints should have been perforated by blood — literally eaten away."

That is one miracle among many I have to be thankful for.

Had I better luck with a general practitioner, I would no doubt have been diagnosed as a hemophiliac much earlier. (Or maybe not. When I read that last sentence to a doctor-friend, she said, "Don't be so sure about that. My husband and I know a couple, both well-trained physicians, who never saw the symptoms of their son's hypoglycemia. When another doctor made the diagnosis, they were mortified.") Without the diagnosis, however, my parents had no real weapon with which to fight my stubborn determination to risk life and limb.

Once the diagnosis came, it was too late. The habit of risk was set. Motocross, skateboarding, domesticated punk: these were constellations by which I navigated my days. I'd read somewhere in Freud that one's life loses interest in direct proportion to its lack of risk. I certainly believed so. When my hemophilia was finally diagnosed, I decided not to let my life be scripted by my doctors no matter how many bleeds I suffered as a result. I raced motocross clandestinely, without my parents' knowing about it, for another year or so. You might say that I was either a "self-actualizing" child or a monster, depending on your point of view.

Much to the delight of my parents, other strategies to "be well" eventually supplemented my earlier, frenetic ambitions. Of these, writing has been the most consistently provocative. While writing is less threatening, physically, than motocross racing or riding a skateboard on my hands, it carries its own considerable risks and gratifications. Writing has played a vital role for me in establishing a psychic equilibrium with hemophilia, an equilibrium that is solid even as it is provisional and ambiguous.

———

A conspiracy of chance and genes deposited me in West Virginia. Chance also conspired to bring about a "spontaneous mutation" in one gene on my X chromosome to give me hemophilia. There was no history of the disease in my family. My mother was not a carrier. (A recessive X-linked disease, hemophilia is almost always passed from a female carrier to her son.) In a fit of random chromosomal dyslexia, the unsuspecting gene could not read the genetic information responsible for coagulation.

"Chance is myself," said Artaud. A troubling notion, and yet what could be more obvious? We know from physicists that chance is at work in the foundation of the atom. We know, too, of course, that we are constructed of atoms. But an abyss lies between our understanding of matter's mercurial hidden life and the affirmation that *our* lives are irradiated through and through by randomness.

For a hemophiliac, trivial events—walking by a table's edge, clapping hands, stepping onto a leaf-obscured or icy curb—are riddled with the chance of a bleed. Once I lifted a gallon of milk in such a way as to break a blood vessel in my elbow. The joint's interior filled with blood until my elbow looked like a steroid-enhanced eggplant.

There are fewer than twenty thousand hemophiliacs in the United States. The odds against any one person's having hemophilia are enormous. The odds against acquiring it through a spontaneous mutation, and not hereditarily, are almost unthinkable. I tried to make sense of chance's role in my life by defying it. I taunted chance, snickered and leered at it, tweaked its nose. My hematologists, not to mention my parents, begged me to stop putting myself in danger as they infused me with clotting factor after I overshot a corner in a motocross race, my bike's foot peg puncturing my calf muscle, or misjudged a skateboard ramp and floated through seized air into the side of a Volkswagen camper.

When John died in 1980, I decided to stop indulging in counterphobia. Of course, I always knew, intellectually, that I could die from a bleed. But John's death made palpable death's absurd immediacy, as though his emaciated body had been blocking the view of my own grave.

Ironically my brother's disease and my own were randomly symmetrical. They were absolutely unrelated, and yet there were days when John's shunt clotted and he needed heparin to get his blood to *stop* coagulating. Meanwhile, I'd start a bleed in a joint and would need factor VIII or cryoprecipitate to get my blood to clot. Literally, what was life to John was death to me. It's as though we underwent a strange, contradictory wash in the gene pool. No doubt, it was utterly bewildering to my mother and father, who without the least preparation brought into the world two children whose chromosomal accidents seemed to mirror a mythology they would act out in life: inverse siblings, the good and the bad brother.

My defiance had included holding out as long as possible during bleeds before getting an infusion of factor VIII. After John died, I decided to redirect the energy behind my defiance and to receive factor VIII at the first suspicion of a bleed. My hematologist and my parents were delighted.

By 1982, when word spread through the hemophilia community that factor VIII concentrate was probably contaminated with HIV, I had received repeated infusions for bleeds into most of my joints. My decision to treat bleeds aggressively had unwittingly increased my likelihood of infection. Indeed, as information about HIV and the blood supply reached the more anxious thickets of the Midwest, it became inconceivable to me that I had not been infected. That I continue to test negative for HIV baffles me to this day.

———————

This book began as a diary I kept while recovering from a serious bleed in 1989. Whenever I start a bleed, I give myself a project. The projects invariably involve writing or reading or simply listening hard to what's going on around me. Past projects have included writing a series of poems about John's life on the dialysis machine (which became the title poem of my second book, *The Brother's Country*); reading the complete works of Owen Barfield, Virginia Woolf, and Woody Allen (not necessarily in that order); writing imaginary conversations with people I will never meet (a repeated favorite); and recording, as unsentimentally and unhysterically as possible, the life of the five senses during a serious bleed. Through this last project, I hoped to learn something about objectivity under duress. I began to understand Stéphane Mallarmé's remark that he could "count the buttons on the hangman's vest," which before had always struck me as unbelievably fatuous.

The point of these projects is to occupy my mind during the coming weeks so that it won't seize on itself, blotting out all light and wonder and possibility. The mind *will* seize on itself, with numbing predictability and consequences; that's a given for a serious bleed. But a project — some engagement of the mind with anything beyond itself — defers that seizure, weakens its grip, shortens its life.

When my mother and father brought to the hospital the scrapbook full of letters and newspaper articles about my world record in clapping, I hadn't thought about that bizarre event in years. But now, with my concentration coming and going within the vagaries of codeine and joint pain, I couldn't stop thinking about it. Why had I done it? How, practically, had I carried it out? What did my parents, and John, *do* with me? What did they do with themselves? How did I avoid a massive bleed in the palms and wrists and forearms?

In the diary I tried to answer these questions and in so doing opened up a rich, clear vein of memory. Indeed, I had (to shift metaphors) come down with memory. Suddenly. Riotously. Memory quickened me, animating my convalescence. I continued writing in the diary after leaving the hospital and during subsequent bleeds.

In *Intoxicated by My Illness,* Anatole Broyard wrote: "My initial experience of illness was as a series of disconnected shocks, and my first instinct was to try to bring it under control by turning it into a narrative." What I wanted to do in the diary was not to "bring it under control" but to articulate the "series of disconnected shocks": the series of events, memories, voices, conversations, prayers, physical tremors and spasms of pain, daydreams, nightmares, all seeming to happen simultaneously — layered upon one another as in a Bach fugue or a rigorous session of channel surfing — that make up the actual experience of surviving a bleed.

Now I've tried to bring the diary itself "under control by turning it into a narrative." Well, not exactly. *Under control* still sounds a bit intrusive to me. Put another way, I hope I've listened carefully to the narratives lurking within the diary. It has been important to include those memories, voices, conversations, and so forth. While they may make this book more a novel than anything else, that's as it should be. There *is* a great deal of invention — of the mind finding ways to make survival sound interesting, convincing, desirable — involved in any trauma and recuperation. I would invoke Wallace Stevens again, who wrote what persons with chronic illnesses know only too well: "The real is the base. But it is only the base." In fact, I've found that what *doesn't* happen is as much a part of the experience of a bleed as what does happen, as oxymoronic as that sounds. Fears, desires, dreams: they are fulfilled or not, but in either case they leave a residue, like the odor of a chrysanthemum that is no longer in the room.

———

There is hemophilia, and there is the "idea" of hemophilia. The former is unalterable. It exists in the world determined by — to use a phrase of Francis Bacon's — the brutality of fact. The latter is slippery. The latter depends upon the hemophiliac. What will my experience of hemophilia be like? Will it cripple my spirit as well as my joints? Will I be able to maneuver between denial on the one hand and self-pity on the other? Answering such questions depends largely on how willing I am to involve my imagination and attention, to be at times outrageous, even crazy — a bad insurance risk.

Hemophilia, in other words, is the base. But it is only the base.

2. SOMETHING RICH AND STRANGE

The trajectory of a bleed and recovery, like that of any illness, is certainly arduous. But it is not only arduous. Jorge Luis Borges, in the preface to a collection of his poems titled *The Unending Rose*, remarked that

> *Going over the proofs of this book, I notice with some distaste that blindness plays a mournful role, which it does not play in my life. Blindness is a confinement, but it is also a liberation, a solitude propitious to invention, a key and an algebra.*

There's so much that I don't know about hemophilia, that I will never know. But I *do* know that each bleed "liberates" me from the hypnosis of daily life. During a bleed, daily life is seen for what it is: a puzzling miracle. During convalescence, I'm inhabited, as never before (it's always "as never before," no matter how recently another bleed occurred), by the instinct to praise, to utter stammering gratitude for being alive.

In the wake of the AIDS debacle, however, I've learned to keep a watchful eye on that instinct to praise. When I am tempted, as I often am, to thank God for having avoided HIV and AIDS, I think at once of a story Primo Levi tells in *Survival in Auschwitz* about the October 1944 "selection." On the day of selection, an SS subaltern judged which Jews would die in the gas chamber during the next few days. When "old Kuhn," one of the men in the camp, was passed over, his neighbor being selected instead, he began praying aloud and swaying back and forth, thanking God that he had not been chosen.

"If I were God," Levi wrote, "I would spit at Kuhn's prayer."

I can well imagine God's spitting at my prayer of thanks for being passed over by AIDS.

In the wake of AIDS, I've resumed motorcycle riding, skateboarding, basketball. I think of these activities now not so much as ways to defy chance but as means to participate in it, listen to it, even — though this will strike many as ludicrous — honor it. When I was convinced I had HIV, the future narrowed to a point. The past expanded and contracted in waves. Only the present was stable. And the present felt like a continent yet to be explored. I resolved to set out across it, to spend my days exuberantly, wonderingly, intimately, with irrational desire. The tightrope balance required to take an off-camber corner at speed, weaving the bike through low, tilted sunlight; kicking up into a handstand on a moving skateboard, watching the vivid world flash by upside down; the body's uncannily timed stretch to block an opponent's layup — to me, these counterphobic talismans suggest there are factors of the blood yet to be enumerated.

And yet, despite the counterphobic impulse that leads me to court significant risk, the image I keep coming back to — the single image that most fully embodies my experience of hemophilia — is one of John shortly before his death.

For a long time I had been asking John to come watch me race motocross. Again and again he refused. Finally he agreed to attend a race at Hidden Hills Raceway in Gallipolis, Ohio — to shut me up, I think, as much as to satisfy his curiosity about his hemophiliac brother's racing a motorcycle across the gouged wilderness.

The road from Charleston to Gallipolis follows the Kanawha River to Point Pleasant, where the Kanawha and Ohio Rivers converge in a vast capital T sunk into bottomland. We passed coal barges drudging through the black water, their wakes spreading across the width of the river and lapping both banks. Before we got to Point Pleasant, it started to rain heavily. Past Gallipolis, just past the farms and the headquarters of Bob Evans Restaurants, we turned off the interstate onto a series of rain-slicked fire roads that led to the track. We were hauling: three times the pickup nearly slid off the road's shoulder.

Eventually we pulled in to the pit area at Hidden Hills. I wondered what John made of the scene: riders tooling the pits, their helmets and shirts off, sideburned, thick arms tattooed and flexing. The smell of Bel-Ray oil and WD-40. The ribbon of track snaking the Ohio landscape. Someone gunning a bike's motor; its spit and cough before going silent. He said nothing.

I knew John would have to wear a plastic bag over his shunt arm to keep out the dust. We were lucky it rained. Dust usually billowed wildly after the start of a race, a huge rolling wave breaking over the hills and shrouding the spectators. Rain would keep the dirt moist and on the track.

Midway through the practice sessions, however, the rain stopped. By the time of the first 100cc moto, dust forced John into the cab of the pickup.

That is the image that attacks me now: John in the truck, windows rolled up, reading a book to pass the time while I kicked up the dust all around him.

———

Though he could not follow the one motocross race he saw in person, John seemed to thrive on my reckless adventures. He told me that he experienced another world through them, a remote and inhospitable world, and I was pleased to introduce him to it. I developed an awareness of living two lives, one superimposed on the other: my own and the phantom life John was not able to lead.

Now that John is dead, he is doing the same for me. In death he underwent, just as Shakespeare said he would, "a sea-change / into something rich and strange."

Into something, yes. But what?

3. THE AMATEUR HEMOPHILIAC

For more than a year now I've assumed this book would end with those last paragraphs.

So why doesn't it?

Well, I'm left with several uncomfortable sensations. I wonder, for example, if I'm not playing into a pathology—a pathology I've worked hard to acknowledge and exorcise — by ending with an image of John. The movement toward health, for me, seems to include ceasing to use John as a measuring stick for my every action. And yet I want very much to articulate the felt pulse of John's absence.

I see.

I'm also uncomfortable with the suggestion that I've *survived* hemophilia once and for all, that I've had my epiphany about the importance of "being well while ill" and that's that.

Don't make me laugh.

I know, I know. Nothing could be further from the truth. In fact, I've noticed that whenever I sense a complacency entering into my relationship with hemophilia —

Your unfinished *relationship with hemophilia.*

Right. Whenever I sense a complacency entering into that relationship, I do something outrageous to stir things up.

Such as?

Remember this past summer? I bought a dirt bike and entered a motocross race for the first time in twenty years.

I was hoping you'd forgotten about it.

How could I? I'd just moved to West Lafayette, Indiana, after spending a year in St. Paul working on this book. Thinking about motocross brought with it a fierce urge to get back out on a track. After about nine months or so of fighting the urge, I decided to give in to it.

Are you a complete idiot?

Was that a rhetorical question? Yes, of course, it was ridiculous, quixotic, idiotic — you name it. After I bought the bike — a Kawasaki KLX 250, which I chose for its user-friendly suspension and power —

I can just see the ad campaign: "Kawasaki: the Choice of Hemophiliacs Everywhere."

After I got the bike, I practiced riding it at motocross tracks around the state of Indiana. I was terrified. Terrified and exhilarated. Of course, I mummified myself with protective gear. I'll tell you, there's nothing like clearing your first double-jump in twenty years. The timing, the momentum approaching the jump —

God help me. Do I have to listen to this?

Hear me out. Actually, the first time I cleared a double-jump, I was so excited that I completely forgot about the sharp right-hand corner immediately following. I cleared the jump, shouted for joy, and overran the corner. The bike sank into the deep sand of the berm. But I'd done it!

Please.

The more I practiced, the faster and more confident I became. Eventually I decided that I would enter the thirty-five-plus class (a thirty-five-year-old is a dinosaur in the world of motocross) at the Fourth of July races at Leisure Time MX

Park in Medaryville, Indiana. I called my friends Joe Bonomo and Amy Newman (both are poets who teach at Northern Illinois University in De Kalb, which is not too far from Medaryville) and asked if they'd like to meet me at the race and serve as my pit crew. I envisioned Joe and Amy giving me crazily literate pit-board signals: "Your cornering, says Aristotle, is a virtue of the practical intellect. Kick butt!" "The apparition of these faces in the crowd; petals on a wet, black Suzuki." "You can't go on, you'll go on." But Joe and Amy already had plans for the Fourth of July, and as it turned out, I was profoundly relieved they weren't there to watch me take what motocrossers call "soil samples."

You mean you crashed?

Only four times. Though *crash* isn't really the word. Remember the tricyclist in *Laugh-In*?

Arte Johnson?

Right. Arte Johnson. Remember how he used to creep along on his tricycle and suddenly topple over? Well, that's the image that best corresponds with my "crashes." During the second lap of practice I fell over and couldn't get the bike started again. So much for fine-tuning my technique. Fortunately I'd ridden on this track a few weeks earlier.

The riders' meeting followed the practice session. The owner of Leisure Time, a kind, hobbled man with a loudspeaker, addressed the assembled riders. "All right now, listen up. I'm supposed to read this here disclaimer to you." He turned his head and coughed. Then he read a macabre text about how motorcycle racing is inherently dangerous; how by entering the premises we acknowledge that we are in potential danger; how we assume all risks of loss, damage, or injury, including paralysis or death.

When the man finished reading the disclaimer, a young rider with a shaved head and a goatee called out, "How many laps you gonna run today, Don [i.e., how many laps per moto, or heat]?"

"I'm not sure," the man said. "I'm thinking, four or five."

"Five!" the young rider shot back. Several riders started chanting, "Five laps! Five laps!"

"Three!" I wanted to shout. "Two!" I didn't.

"The racing's over by the fourth lap," the man said into the loudspeaker. "What difference does a lap make?"

"Five laps! Five laps!"

"Fine by me," the man said, and then he read the order of the races. The thirty-five-plus class would be the sixth race.

It just occurred to me to ask what Carrie thought of all this.

Believe it or not, she encouraged me to race. Or rather, she encouraged me to follow the rebellious urge that racing embodied. I should probably mention, though, that Carrie and I were no longer married at that point. We were divorced in 1994.

Hmmm. In the wake of divorce you needed to convince yourself that you weren't a relic? What happened between you and Carrie?

I don't mean to dodge your questions but I do want to bracket them for a minute. I'll come back to them, I promise. When I pulled up to the starting gate before the first moto, I thought, *My God! I'm actually doing this. I'm not a kid anymore and I'm actually doing this. Why am I doing this? Isn't there some other activity that perhaps simulates the danger and rebellion I apparently need to act out, but does so without threatening my life?*

And I realized that I was doing it for two reasons. I was about to race motocross again because I needed to affirm that I was still an amateur hemophiliac, that I hadn't turned pro. I was worried about a shift in my relationship with the disease. While writing poems had never had this effect on me (quite the opposite, in fact), writing this memoir has encouraged me to think of hemophilia as something I've *transcended*. Hemophilia hasn't defeated *me*. After all, here I am outwitting it, writing about it in a memoir that Little, Brown (a publisher I've adored since I was a kid because it published Peter De Vries) is going to publish. My implied stance seems to be: I fought the chromosomal law and I won.

Fat chance.

Exactly. While writing this book, I was continually tempted to take myself seriously as a "hemophiliac," whatever that is.

What do you mean, "whatever that is"? Surely a hemophiliac is someone with hemophilia.

Of course that's true — as far as it goes. It just doesn't go far enough. My point is that it's up to each person with hemophilia to define what hemophilia means. It's up to me to decide what — who — a hemophiliac is. And I hope never to figure it out. Our culture urges people with chronic illnesses to resolve rich tensions that to my mind are better left unresolved. That motocross race in Medaryville was a way of making sure I was still involved in a flawed, ongoing, *human* relationship.

So what happened? How'd you do?

Well, I crashed, or toppled over, twice in the first moto and didn't finish. In the second moto I toppled over right in front of the grandstand, but at least I was able to get up in time to finish.

The only thing I can think to do is shake my head.

You're not wrong to do so.

You said there was a second reason you entered that race.

Yes. I think it has to do with the lingering effect of AIDS. Imagine AIDS as an enormous motocross race in which every racer's throttle is stuck wide open. Nine out of ten hemophiliacs who had repeated infusions between 1978 and 1985 crash horribly. The one out of ten who doesn't crash rides past one unthinkable, deadly scene after another. He's not thinking, *Will I crash?* He's thinking, *When will I crash?* The trick is to remain in the race without having your identity re-volve around the fact that you are a racer who hasn't crashed yet. The trick is to remain in the race because you love racing. Eventually you seem to be racing on a different track from the other riders — a parallel track that never intersects theirs. But you're not. You're on the same track, and you keep racing and racing.

You're saying you raced at Medaryville in order to act out the little parable you just told me?

I've never thought to put it that way, but yes, partly. I raced in order to see if I still loved racing.

And do you?

Yes, metaphorically. But not literally!

I'm confused. Does that mean you will or will not race mo-tocross again?

It means I will not — at least, not in the near future. There's always the fifty-plus class to think about later. The truth is, though, I was bored by speed. I'd forgotten that speed was the name of the game. It was shocking to realize the degree to which sharing a nuanced and precise language — replete with terms like *holeshots, whoop-de-doos, can-cans, endos, cross-ups, heel clickers,* and so forth — informed, maybe even cre-ated, the pleasures of motocross. Now I was a thirty-five-year-old crazed bleeder jock cruising around Indiana's motocross tracks without a group of buddies to talk the talk with. I'd always remembered motocross as a solitary soul-making experience. It turns out it was a profoundly social soul-making experience. Lacking the social element, racing proved to be surprisingly empty of significance. In fact, writ-ing poems gives me the sensation of having more at risk, and more significantly, than I did during that motocross race. Does that make sense?

No.

Well, the stakes seem to be higher, the sense of adventure greater, when working on a poem. You never know what you're doing. In motocross you make the same moves over and over, lap after lap. Don't get me wrong. I'm not saying motocross is safer. I'm saying it *feels* riskier to write a poem when you're writing within a spirit of openness and receptivity. So. To answer your question, I'll keep my ratty old street bike to bop around town on, but I don't plan on racing again anytime soon.

All right. Now tell me what happened with Carrie.

While I was writing this book, I often asked myself whether hemophilia had anything to do with our divorce. And I could never come to a conclusion. So the other day I called Carrie and asked her what she thought.

You did?

Why not? Without hesitating, Carrie said, "I don't think hemophilia had anything to do with our divorce. But I think hemophilia has a lot to do with your compulsion to write, and *that* sure had a lot to do with our divorce." Clear-eyed Carrie. God love her. Thinking back, it's probable that our troubles started when I decided I wasn't up to the challenges of having children at the same time that Carrie decided she wanted them. But who's to say my decision was based on the fact of my hemophilia? I knew of hemophiliacs who embraced parenthood (though I didn't know any of them personally). We could have adopted children, if my only concern was the moral implications of passing on the dyslexic gene on my X chromosome. As Carrie said, my need to spend hour after hour pushing words around surely made me a less-than-sterling husband. Beyond that, though, I believe our divorce had to do with a collision of circumstances that lie outside the scope of this book. I'm grateful that Carrie and I remain close friends, and I don't want to say anything that would betray that friendship. Fair enough?

Fair enough.

Enough said?

Enough said.

GUINNESS SUPERLATIVES LIMITED
2 Cecil Court, London Road
Enfield, Middlesex EN2 6DJ
Telephone: 01 366 4551
Telegrams and cables: Mostest Enfield

Mr H Raymond Andrews Jr
1714 Rolling Hills Circle
Charleston
West Virginia 25314
USA

9 May 1973

Dear Mr Andrews:

I apologise for the delay in replying to your letter due to a longish absence away from my desk in the US and subsequently on the continent.

I think that the authentification on the new hand clapping duration record is now satisfactory.

We shall be revising material for a new edition during this summer, and I only hope that the deed of last November is not overtaken in the interim.

With all best wishes.

Yours sincerely,
NORRIS D McWHIRTER
Editor

ACKNOWLEDGMENTS

Anyone who has read this far knows what a debt I owe to Ray and Alice Andrews, my good-humored, long-suffering parents. I am grateful beyond words for their abiding love and support.

In Gordon Kato I have — thanks to Keith Taylor — the most supportive and intelligent agent imaginable. Time and again, when I was convinced that I had no business (no talent, no inner resources, etc.) writing this book, Gordon found ways to convince me otherwise. His faith in this project made it possible.

I thank my editors at Little, Brown, Geoffrey Kloske and Jordan Pavlin, for their patience, their generosity of spirit, their sanity, and their advocacy of this book. I also thank Stephen Lamont, whose meticulous copyediting improved the book considerably.

David Lazar answered with great patience my endless questions about the possibilities of creative nonfiction, helping me find ways to conjure up this book.

Many years ago, the poet Priscilla Sneff introduced me to *Journey,* Robert and Suzanne Massie's memoir of raising a son with hemophilia, and suggested that writing about this aspect of my experience might be a valuable endeavor. Many other friends and loved ones helped me finish this book. I would like especially to acknowledge the invaluable help given me by Carrie Andrews, Emily Worden-Meuleman and Dave Meuleman, Julie Trachtenberg, Anne MacDonald, Charles Wright, Wayne Dodd and Joyce Barlow Dodd and the Doddo Writers' Colony, Brian Kiteley and Cynthia Coburn, Mark

Shelton, Joe Bonomo and Amy Newman, Alyson Hagy, Alyce Miller, Caryn Kunkle, Mike Chitwood, Tony Crunk, Janet Holmes and Al Greenberg, Richard Solly, Mary Bisbee, Bill Lychack, Georgia Newman, Janet Abrahm, and Katie Watson. I send a hearty bear hug to my co-conspirators at *Mathematical Reviews,* especially Paula Shanks and the late D. J. Kimball.

I am also grateful to my colleagues in the creative writing program at Purdue University—Marianne Boruch, Patricia Henley, Neil Myers, and Chuck Wachtel—for granting me time off from teaching to complete this book.

Finally, I would not have lived to write this book were it not for the careful ministrations of Dr. Robert Roddy and Jennifer Nash-Wright and the staff at McCafferty, Roddy and Associates in St. Paul, Minnesota. To them, and to the many physicians who have worked with me (rarely a rewarding assignment) over the years, my profound thanks.